sex

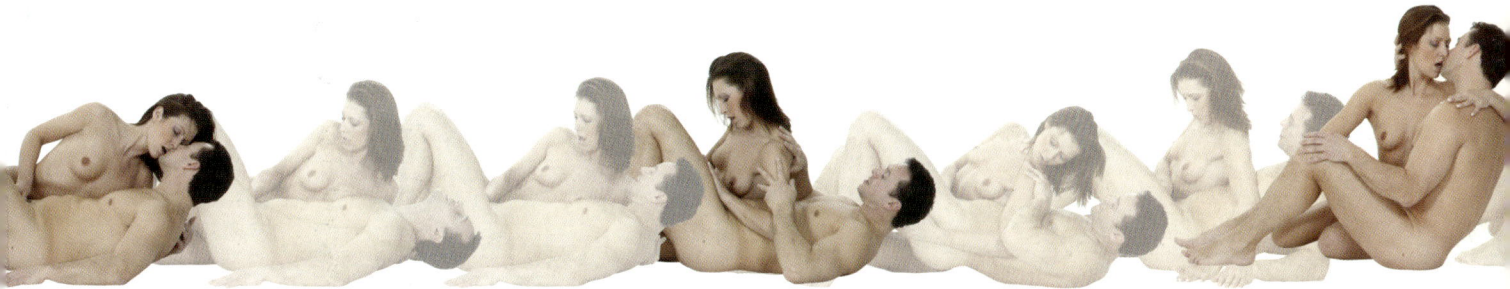

a *flow*motion™ title

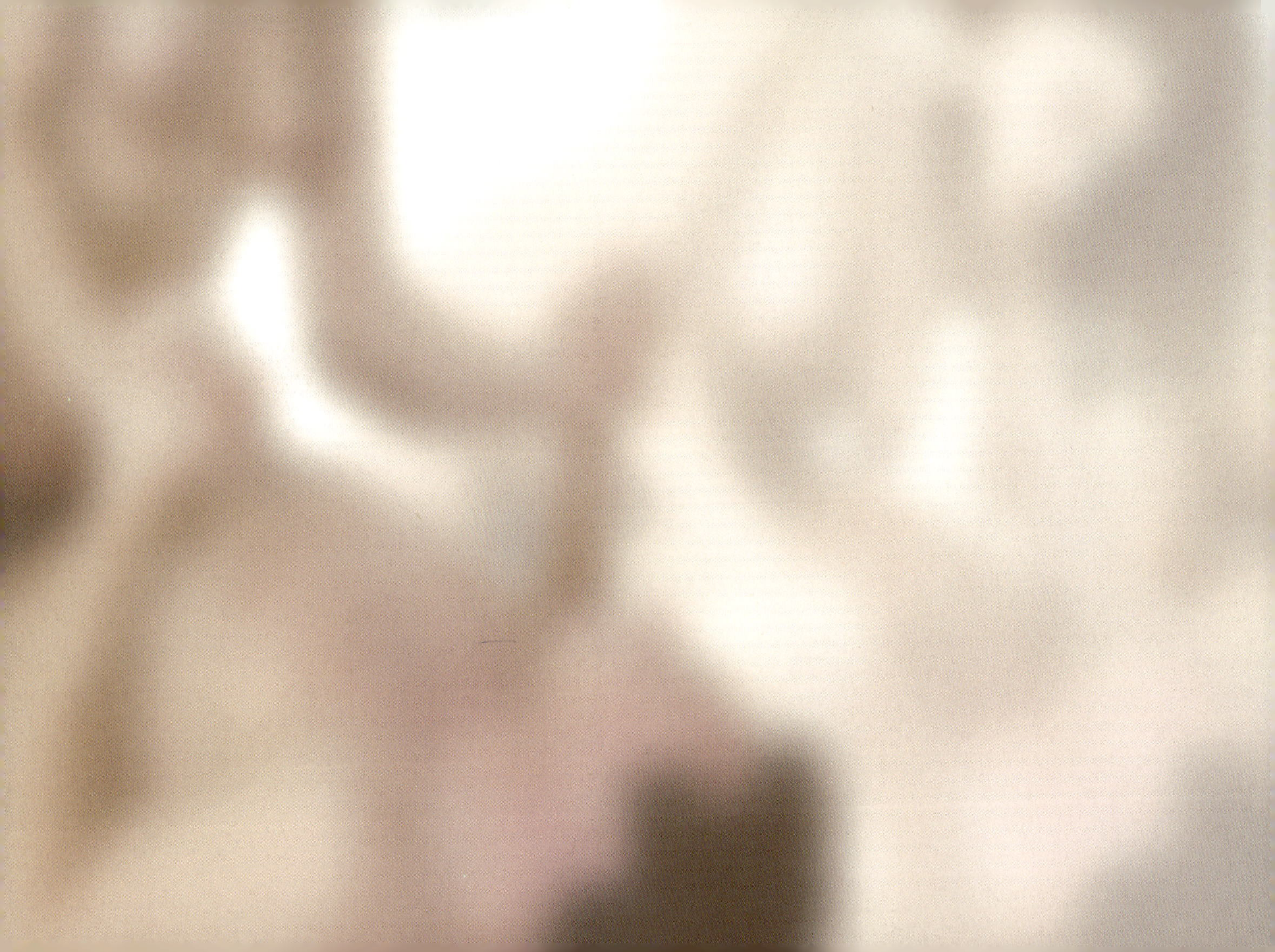

sex

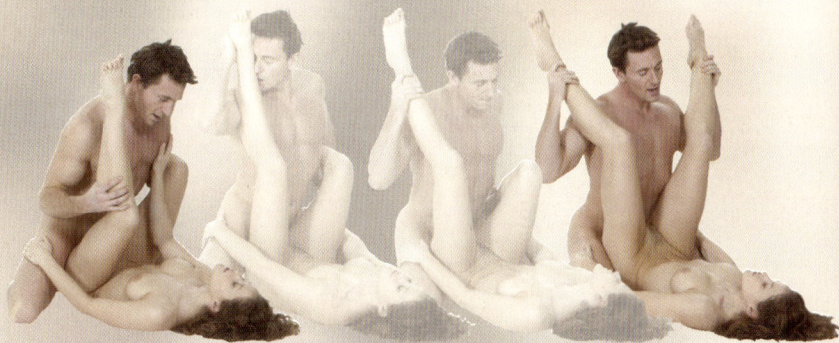

richard craze

Sterling Publishing Co., Inc.

New York

Created and conceived by
Axis Publishing Limited
8c Accommodation Road
London NW11 8ED
www.axispublishing.co.uk

Creative Director: Siân Keogh
Editorial Director: Brian Burns
Project Designer: Axis Design Editions
Managing Editor: Conor Kilgallon
Production Controller: Juliet Brown
Photographer: Mike Good

Library of Congress Cataloging-in-Publication Data
Available

10 9 8 7 6 5 4 3 2 1

Published in 2003 by Sterling Publishing Co., Inc.
387 Park Avenue South, New York, NY 10016
Text and images © Axis Publishing Limited 2003
Distributed in Canada by Sterling Publishing
C/o Canadian Manda Group,
One Atlantic Avenue, Suite 105
Toronto, Ontario, Canada, M6K 3E7

ISBN 1–4027–0902–1

Printed by Star Standard (Pte) Limited

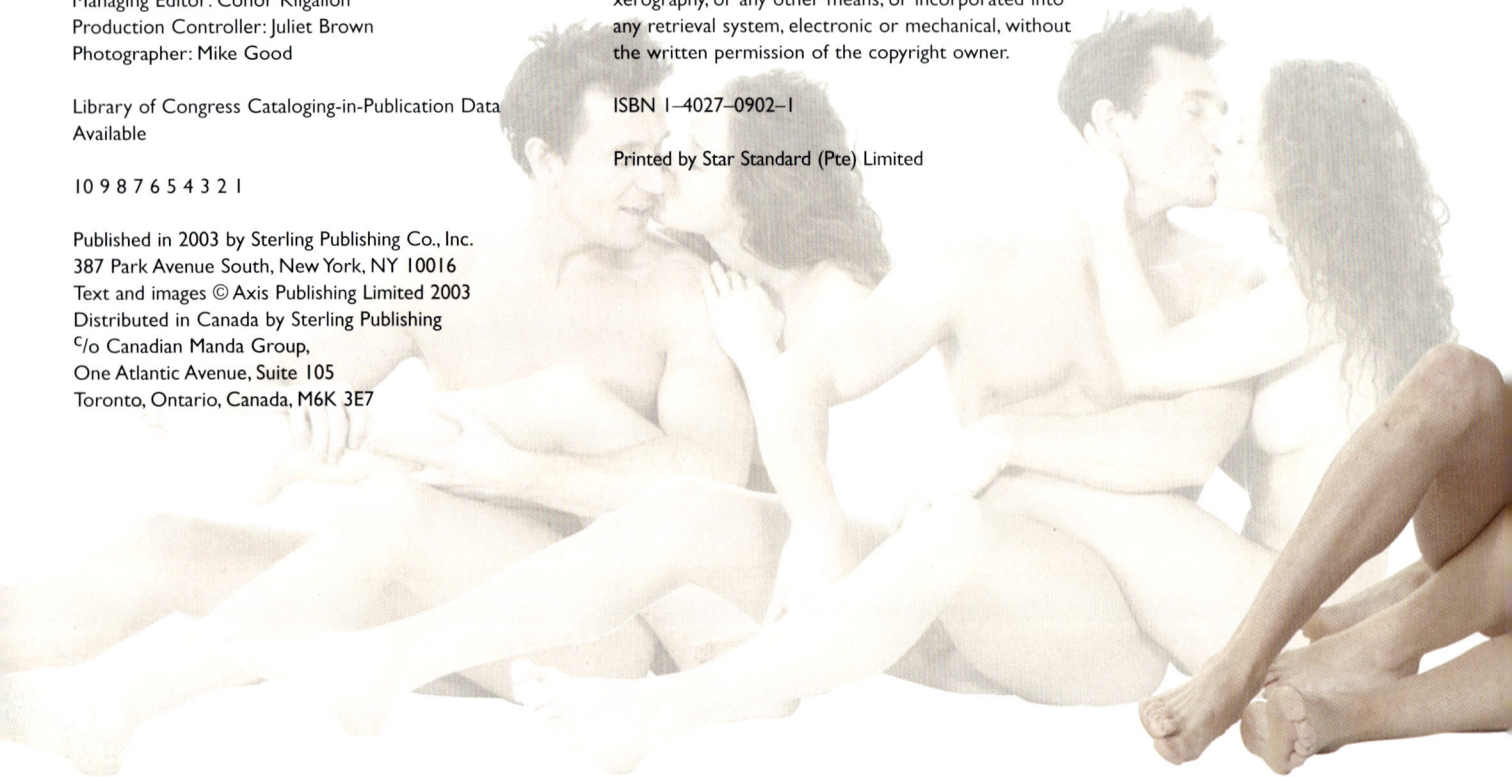

a *flow*MOTION™ title

sex

contents

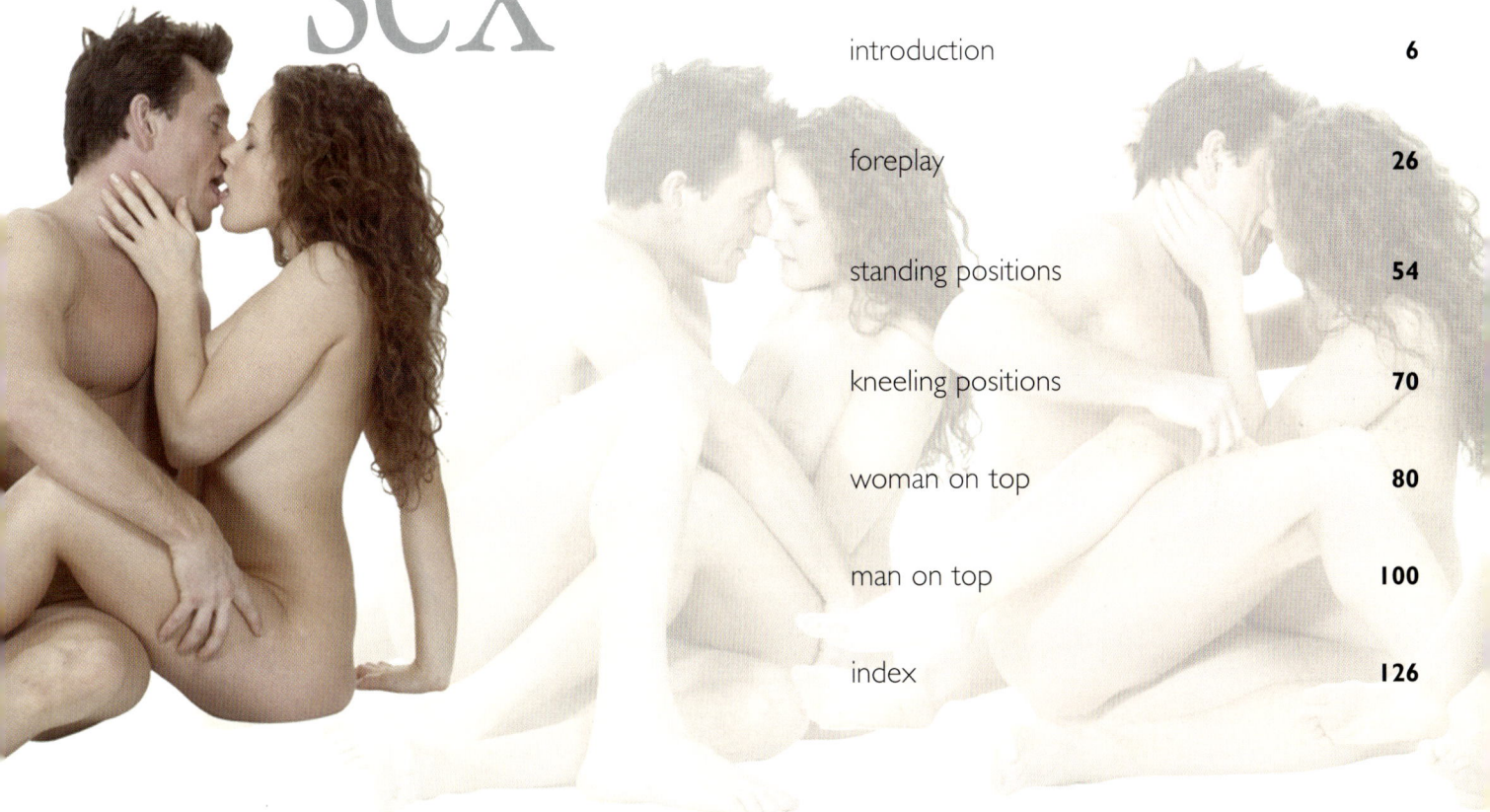

setting the scene

Flowmotion Sex introduces you to a whole new concept of sex book—one where you can really see how to do it, improve it, enhance it, and enjoy it more. We all have sex, so doing it better must be a good thing.

   We live in a time when sex is everywhere. It is in newspapers, magazines, and television programs—it is even used to sell cars. But the sex in this book is completely different. It allows you to see exactly how two lovers come together, showing how easy some of the traditional positions are. This will give you the impetus and the enthusiasm to try new things, to experiment, and be open to new experiences.

driving and sex

There are two things that no one will ever admit to—being a bad driver or being a poor lover. Can you imagine anyone ever announcing, "I'm a hopeless driver," or "I've never quite mastered the lovemaking thing." No one ever admits to needing to learn more. That's why this book really helps because it shows us all how to improve without ever having to admit publicly that we needed to in the first place.

what's in it for you

There are no basic biology lessons in this book—it assumes you know your way around your own body pretty well, know what all the parts are called and what they do. It also assumes that you are in a stable and loving

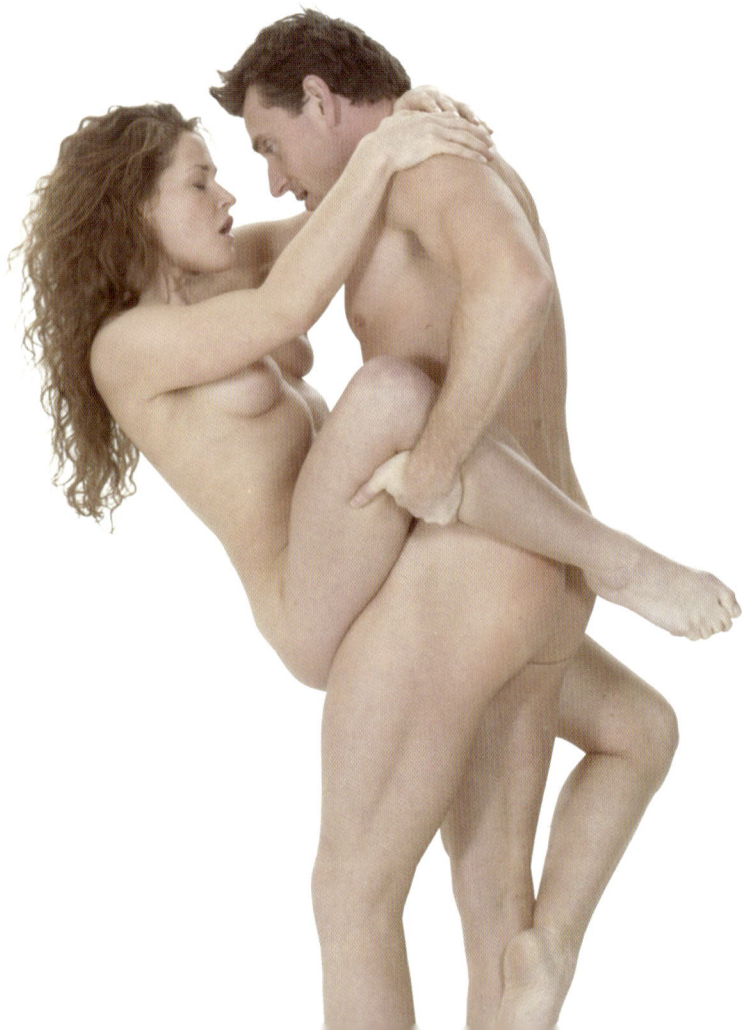

relationship—this book isn't for those who like one-night stands or for those seeking casual sex.

The only way to improve our sexual relationships is to work at them. We have to put in effort, time, thought, and care. So subjects such as getting in the mood, setting the scene, seducing your lover, erotic undressing, foreplay, food play, erogenous zones, flirting, erotic kissing, and the best techniques of oral sex are all covered. It also looks at what happens not only before and during sex but also after sex and how to bathe in the warm glow and satisfaction with your partner.

getting in the mood

If you turn to your lover and blatantly say, "Sex tonight?" the chances are the answer will be "no." That's easy enough to predict. You have to create the mood first, set the scene, perhaps through seductive lighting and good decor. You have to tidy the bedroom first, light some candles, burn a little incense. The more time and effort you put in, the greater the rewards. Sex is like any other activity. You wouldn't expect to go skydiving without first having booked the plane, packed your parachute, and put on your jump suit. Good sex might happen at the end of the day, but the preparation starts the minute you wake up; the long, slow, lingering kiss, saying "good morning, I love you," and the breakfast in bed are all seduction techniques designed to light fires and stimulate desire.

Sex is more than just two bodies coming together in physical harmony. It is also an intimate meeting of minds, emotions, and spirits.

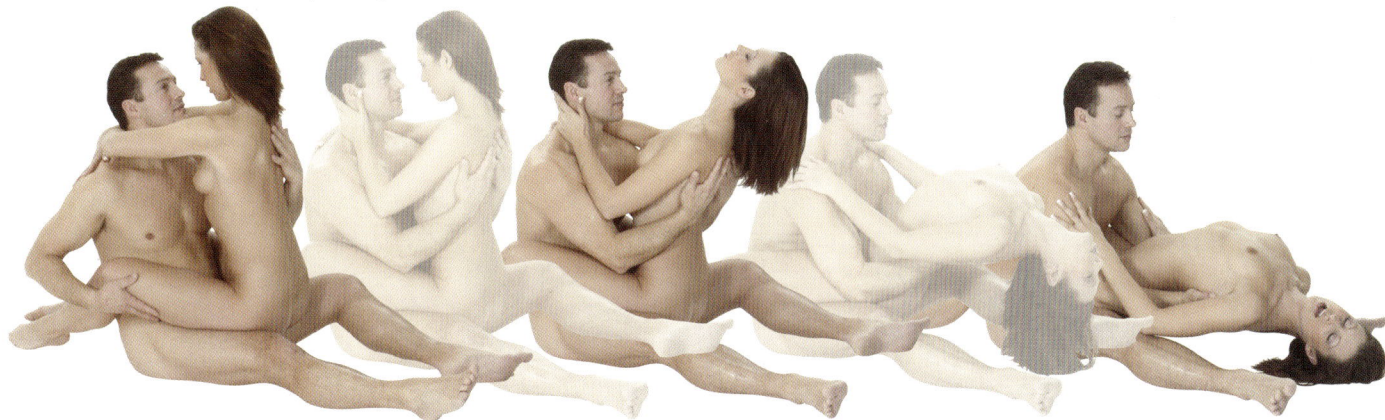

turn-ons I

erotic undressing

Slowly exposing your body to your lover is a skill. There may be times when ripping off your clothes in a frenzied passion is appropriate, but more often it is the slow removing of clothing that turns them on, warms their blood, and kindles their lust. You don't have to be a stripper but you can be subtle, teasing, evocative, and erotic. It's not what you take off but how you take it off that is important. Allowing a little glimpse of something forbidden is much more erotic than a blatant, full-on show. And taking off your clothes is not just a visual thing, but is audio and tactile as well—the sound of zippers being undone and the feel of silk on bare skin all contribute.

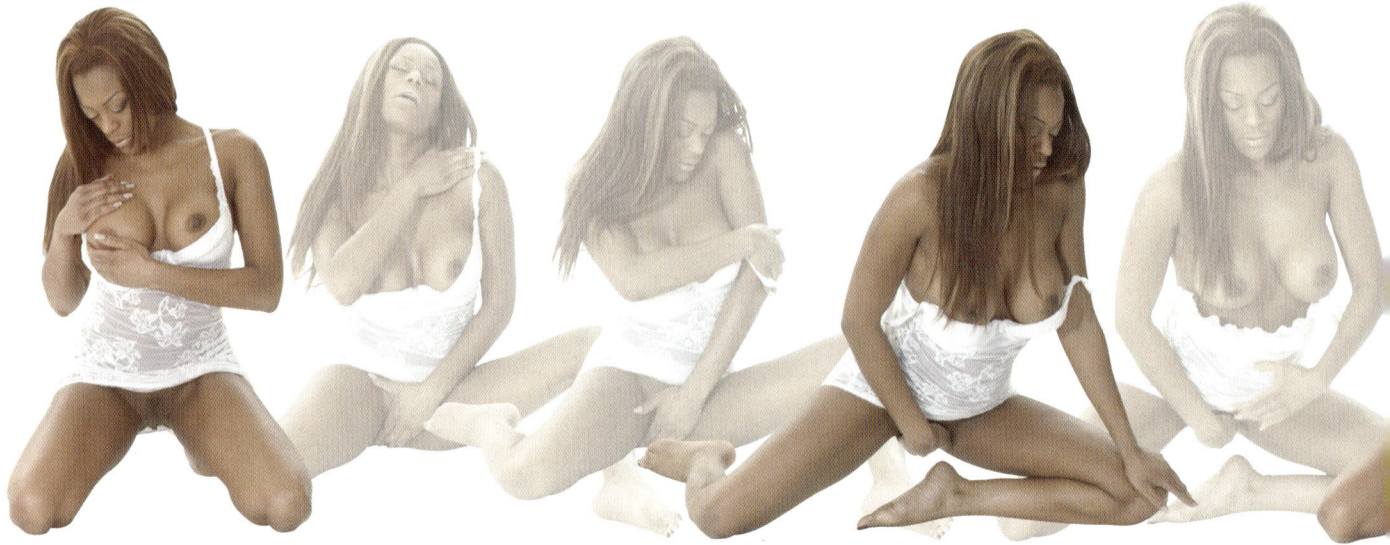

It seems from the research done into the subject that men and women react differently to visual stimulation. Men get turned on by more uninhibited and explicit displays, whereas women often want subtlety and delicacy. The skillful lover works with this information and knows how to turn their lover on merely by undressing in the right way. Always remember that what is not revealed, kept hidden, is often sexier than what is on show. This means keeping something back to tease your lover.

There are, however, some unwritten rules to be aware of; for example, never take off your pants before your socks.

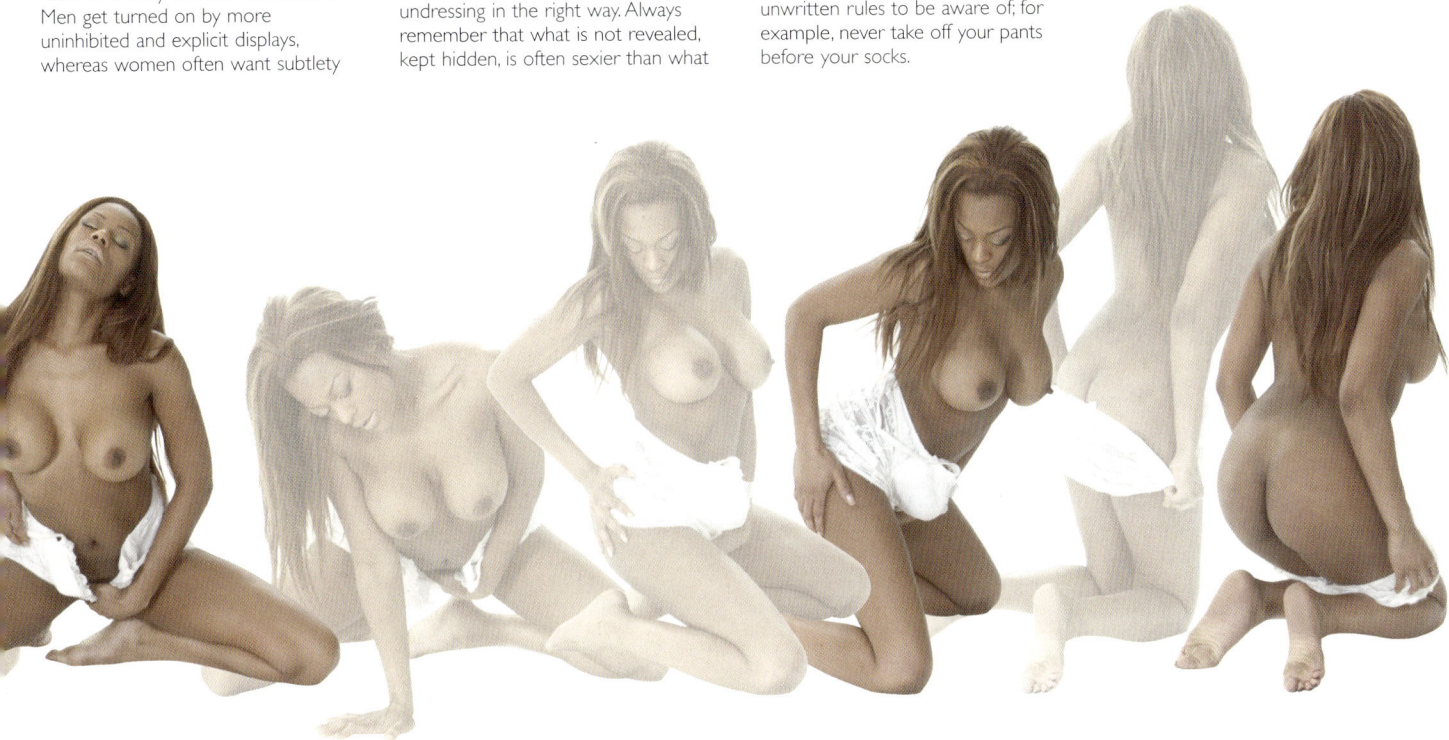

If you are masturbating in front of your lover remember that you aren't just turning yourself on, but your lover as well. With this in mind, you can act out your wildest fantasies, be vocal and very visual. So how you masturbate in private and how you masturbate in front of your lover should be two quite different things. You can be daring, wild, and sexy. Your lover will adore it, and it is very erotic and arousing to act out your fantasies.

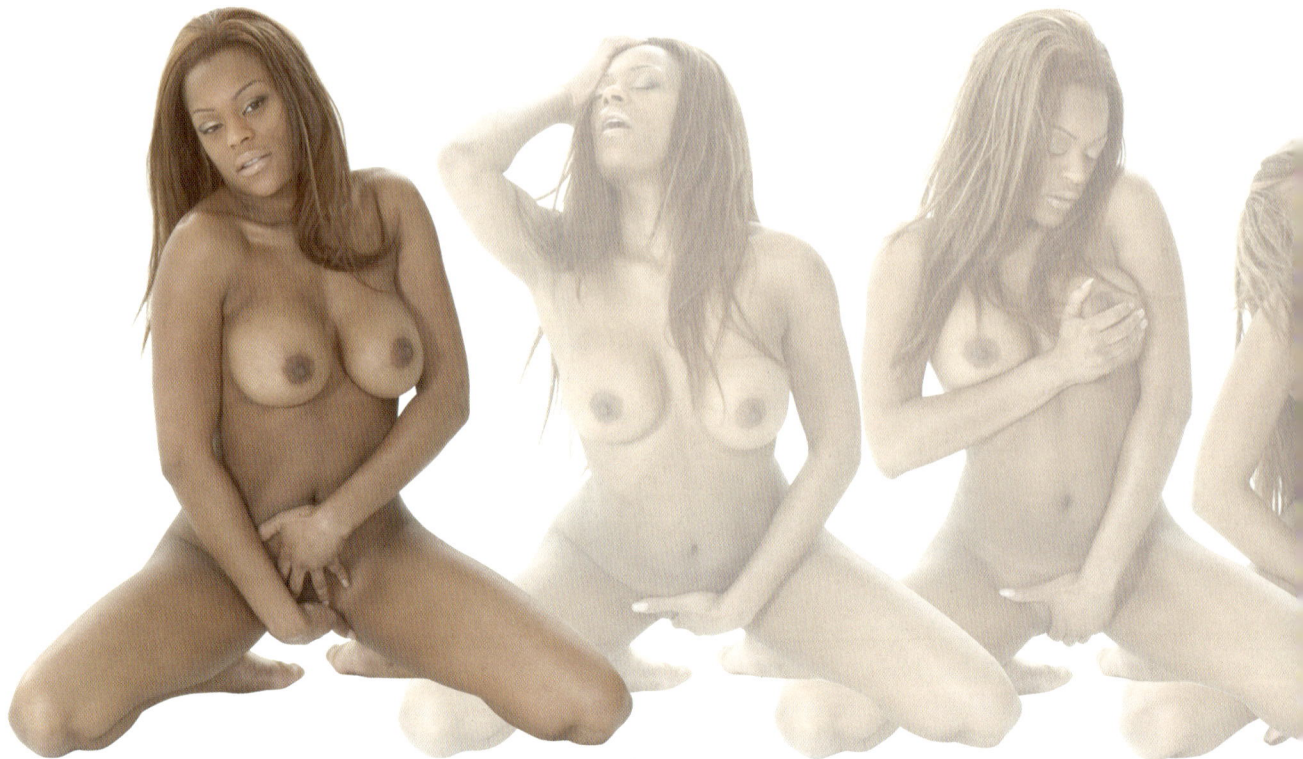

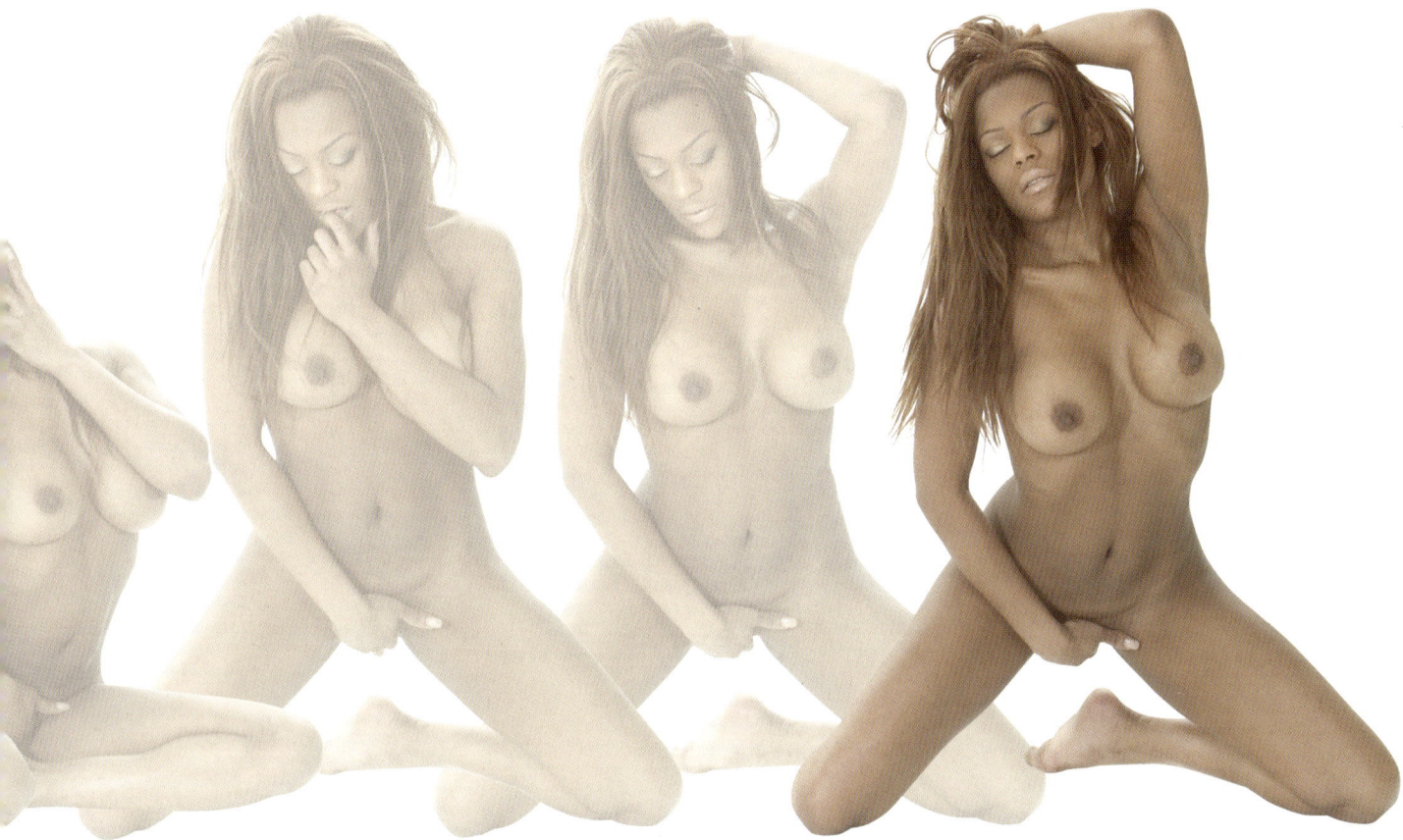

turn-ons II

sex and food

There is nothing more erotic than combining sex and food. Imagine the feel of a freshly bitten strawberry rubbed over your naked body while your lover licks wine from your lips. Why only imagine it? Why not try it this instant? Any food you use during sex as an erotic aid needs to be delicious, tactile, and luscious. We're talking about ice cream, strawberries, wine, champagne, honey, chocolate, yogurt, peaches, bananas, oysters, olives, and more chocolate. We are not talking about hamburgers or french fries, or cups of tea or cabbage. Think slippery. Think luxury. Think moist.

erogenous zones

Good sex isn't just about intercourse. That might be the main course, but the appetizer and the dessert are the erogenous zones. Really good lovers are the ones who spend a great deal of time just paying attention to all

Feeding your lover is very sexy. But you have to choose the right foods—strawberries are sexy, a cup of tea isn't.

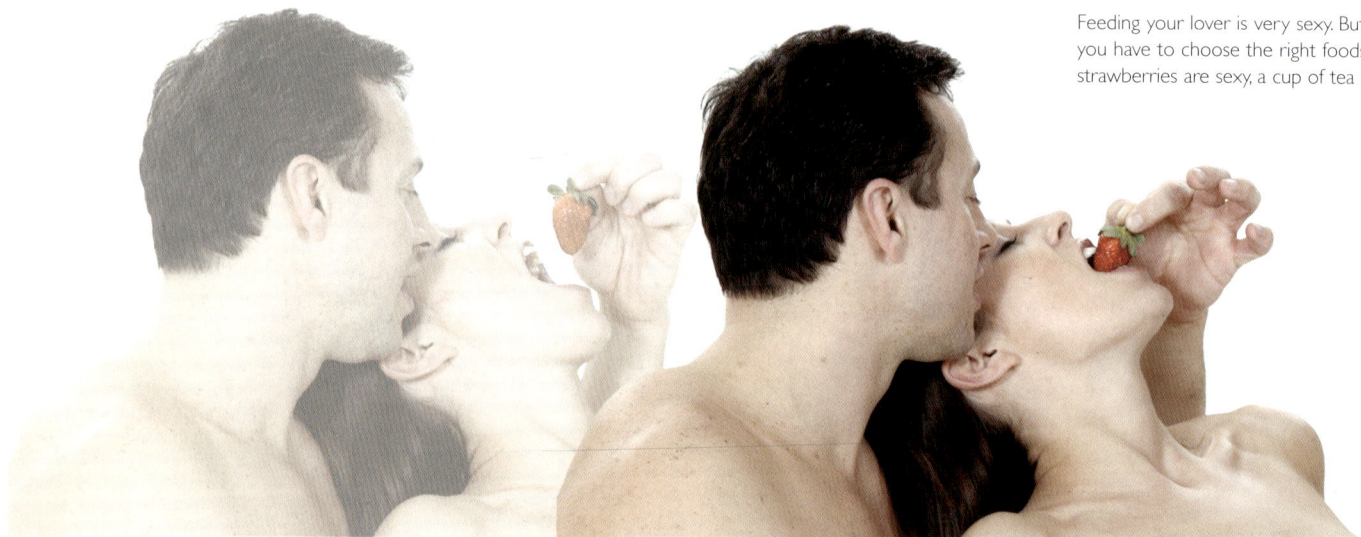

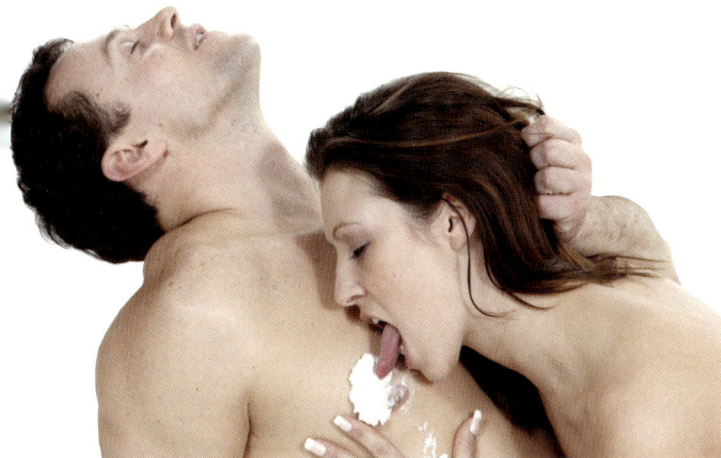

those bits that other, lesser lovers ignore—the armpits, the nipples, the tiny folds in the crook of the elbow, the back of the neck, the hollow by the collarbone, the spaces between the fingers, the backs of the hands, the crooks of the knees, the belly button, the chin, and the eyelids. These are all erogenous zones. These are all sensitive, electric places where licking, sucking, and nibbling have a major effect. These areas are erotic and cry out for attention. Ignore the genitals and concentrate on these lesser areas and your ability as a lover will increase dramatically.

physical flirting

There is flirting—using your eyes and voice to seduce your lover—and there is physical flirting, which can be used to devastating effect during sex. Physical flirting is touching yourself for your lover, teasing, not letting them

NEW SENSATIONS

You can use various techniques during foreplay to make sure your lover stays excited during the whole lovemaking experience. One way of doing this is to heighten the sensory experience by not allowing your lover to know exactly what to expect—or quite when to expect it. Playing with hot and cold sensations is a good way of adding this new dimension to your foreplay.

HOT AND COLD—FOR HIM

Ice cubes are ideal for creating the cold sensation. During oral sex, the woman can pop an ice cube into her mouth and, using her tongue, swirl it around the head of her lover's penis, and see what reactions she gets. But she must be careful not to leave the ice cube on the head of his penis for too long.

A sip of coffee is good for producing a hot sensation, but again, she must be careful not to make it too hot. Alternating between the heat of the coffee and the cold of the ice is an unusual and exciting sensation for most men when they are enjoying fellatio.

HOT AND COLD—FOR HER

The man giving his partner oral sex can also experiment with ice cubes and hot coffee. He can let his tongue chill on the ice and then lick her clitoris; then replace that sensation with one of a hot tongue, heated by the coffee.

He can also hold an ice cube in his mouth, letting it rest on her skin intermittently as he licks her. As well as providing lots of lovely icy sensations, it also generates lots of moisture as the ice melts, increasing the sensitivity of her skin.

EROGENOUS ZONES: HERS

EYELIDS AND EARS

The whole of a woman's face is an erogenous zone. Just taking a woman's face in your hands is often enough to turn her on. Then try licking her eyelids or nibbling on her earlobe.

NECK

Stroking and caressing the neck from behind and licking and scratching the back is very arousing for many women.

BELLY BUTTON

Licking and nibbling this area can be very pleasurable, but this is a sensitive area so take care and be prepared to stop.

NIPPLES

Nipples can be so sensitive that some women can reach orgasm just by having them sucked. Most can't, but licking and massaging them is very arousing.

INSIDE THE ELBOWS

Licking here can make your lover squirm and get turned on. On the other hand, they may just find it unbearably ticklish.

ARMPITS

Some women find their armpits very sensitive and erotic. Experiment to see what your lover thinks.

ASK OR EXPLORE

Explore her entire body with your tongue, your lips, and your fingertips. You'll quickly know which bits are erogenous and which are merely ticklish.

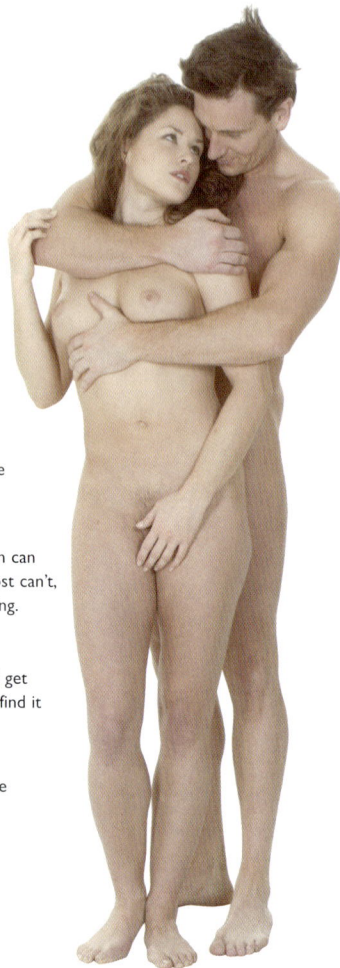

EROGENOUS ZONES: HIS

EYELIDS AND EARS

Some men love having their eyelids licked and their earlobes nibbled.

NECK

Most men find that their necks, backs, and shoulders aren't particularly sensitive.

PUBIC AREA

Try gently scratching around his pubic area and pulling and tugging lightly on his pubic hair. It can drive him wild.

PERINEUM

Most men have a very sensitive perineum (the area of skin between testicles and anus) and love having it scratched lightly. Try playing with his penis at the same time.

NIPPLES

A lot of men have very sensitive nipples and enjoy having them tweaked and sucked. In fact, some men's nipples are so sensitive that they need them to be stroked and pinched to help them acheive a much more intense orgasm.

ASK OR EXPLORE

Try exploring his whole body with your tongue, your lips, and your fingers. The pubic area is, naturally, one area where he is truly sensitive.

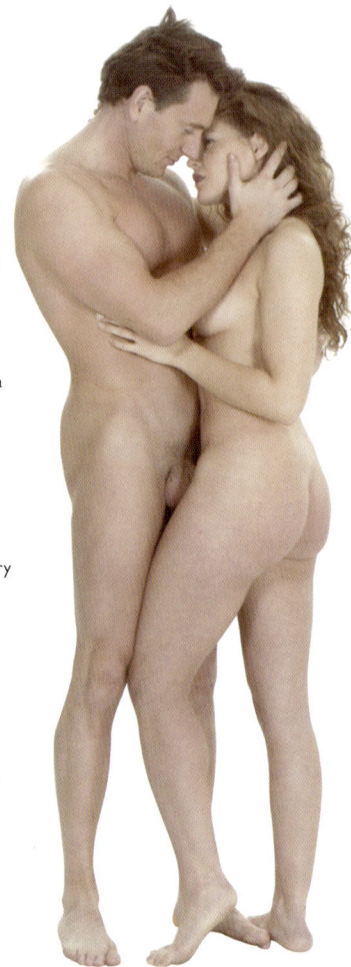

touch, holding back, holding out, turning them on by turning yourself on, putting on a show for their sexual pleasure. If you are comfortable touching yourself, it shows your lover how relaxed and confident you are. There is nothing better than a lover who is totally at home with their own body. It allows your partner to feel relaxed as well. It gives them permission to be wild and wanton, sexy, and liberated. If you are shy, then often the opposite applies, and your lover will feel embarrassed, reticent, and awkward.

erotic kissing

Kissing is the most erotic act we can perform with another human being. In China, kissing is regarded as so erotic that it is not performed in public. Good kissing takes time and practice; the nibbling on lips, the sucking on

tongues, the pressure of lips, the sounds, the moistness, the hands being used to hold your lover's face as you kiss them deeply and slowly.

delaying orgasm

Good sex is a time-consuming activity. The trouble for many men is that they feel they need to rush to orgasm to satisfy their desires, so sex is over too quickly, leaving a partner unsatisfied and disappointed. Good lovers

Time spent kissing usually means better sex and orgasms. Experienced lovers knows this and spend plenty of time kissing before, during, and after sex.

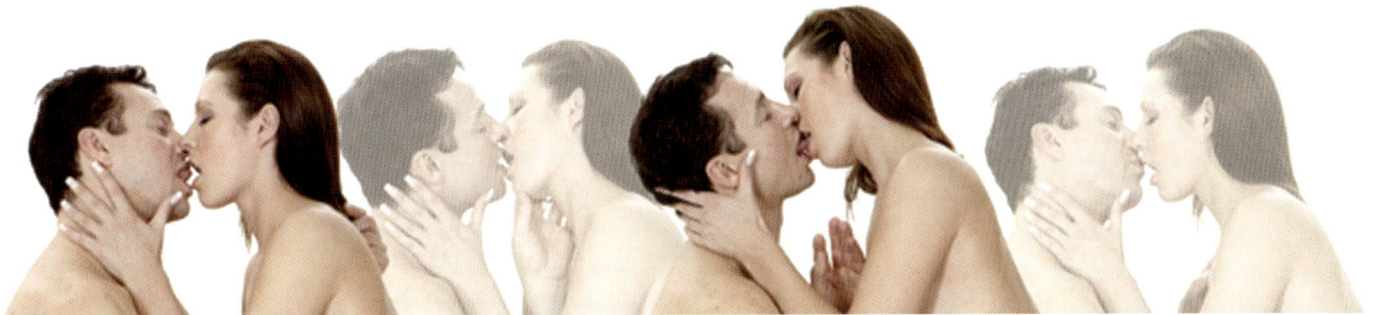

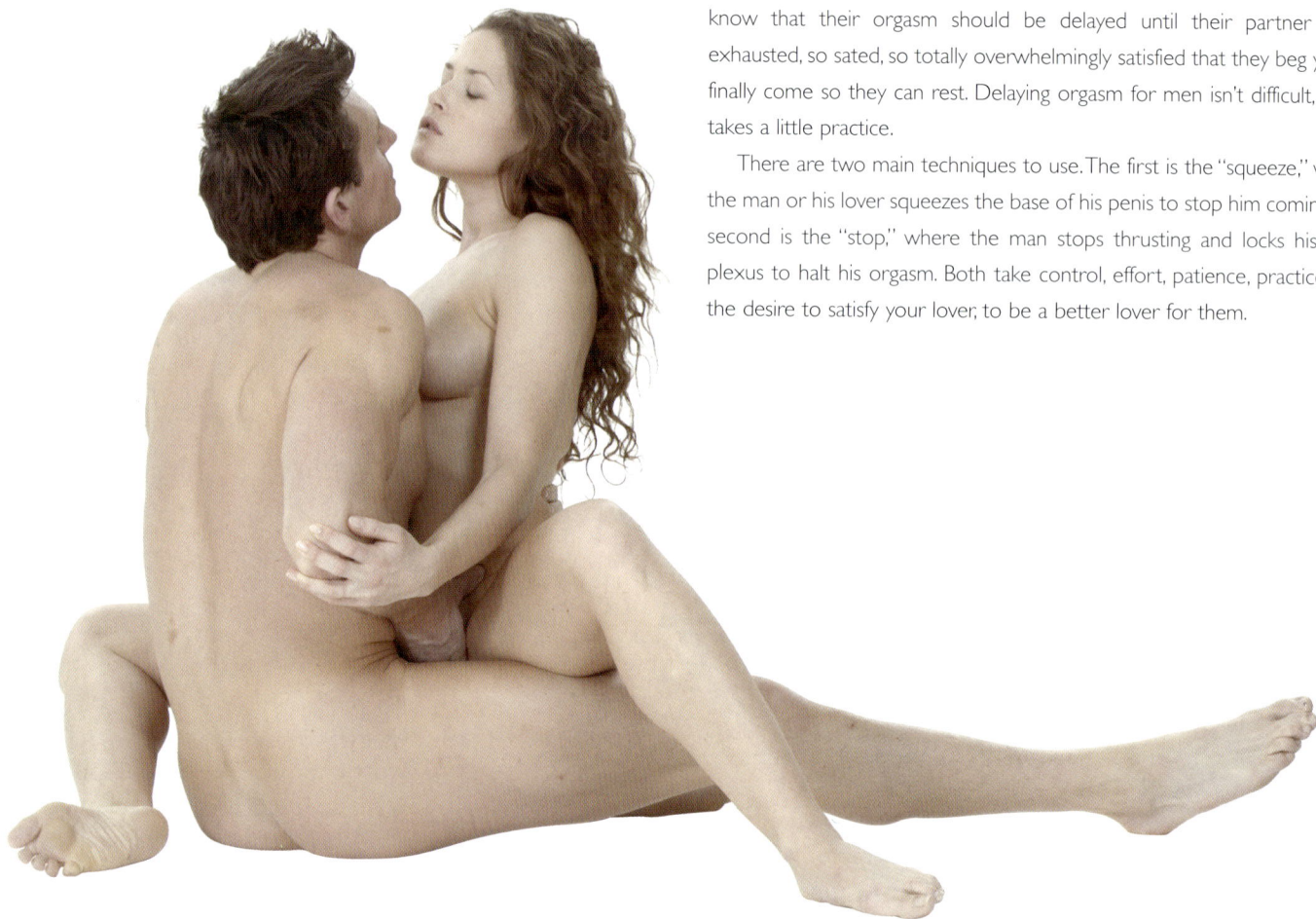

know that their orgasm should be delayed until their partner is so exhausted, so sated, so totally overwhelmingly satisfied that they beg you to finally come so they can rest. Delaying orgasm for men isn't difficult, it just takes a little practice.

There are two main techniques to use. The first is the "squeeze," where the man or his lover squeezes the base of his penis to stop him coming. The second is the "stop," where the man stops thrusting and locks his solar plexus to halt his orgasm. Both take control, effort, patience, practice, and the desire to satisfy your lover; to be a better lover for them.

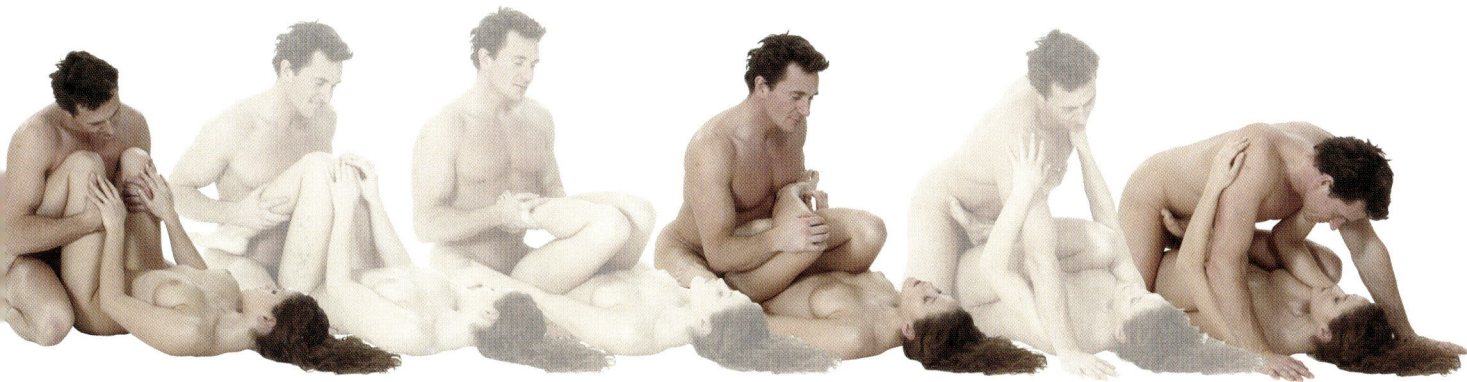

pelvic floor exercises

In the same way that a man wanting to be a good lover will learn how to delay his orgasm, so a woman who wants to be a better lover should pay attention to her pelvic floor exercises. These are specifically designed to tighten her grip on her lover's penis by making her vaginal muscles stronger and more powerful. Locating the pubococcygeus (PC) muscle is easy—you can use it stop the flow of urine when on the toilet. The muscle that performs this task is the correct one to practice squeezing and tightening when not urinating. Performed often enough, this exercise tightens the vaginal muscles very well. This not only makes you a better lover but also increases and improves vaginal control after childbirth.

Sex is a skill that can be learned like any other. Have fun improving as you practice with your lover. You don't have to fumble in the dark.

the right words

Before you read further, a quick note on the language used. No proper Latin terms are used since these risk sounding too medical. No slang appears either, since this can be offensive. Nor are childish words used since these risk sounding trite and coy. Choosing the right language for this subject can be difficult, so words and terms that sound wholesome but sexy, inoffensive but grown up, and proper but not too medical, appear.

limits and boundaries

safe sex

The only truly safe sex is two people having sex with themselves in separate rooms. Otherwise, all sexual contact carries some kind of risk. It might be the risk of sexually transmitted diseases, Aids, unwanted pregnancies, emotional disappointment, unmet expectations, or just plain frustration. We all know what we must do to practice safe sex and avoid unwanted pregnancies and Aids—wear a condom. This book is for couples who know each other well so that transmitting sexual diseases shouldn't be an issue.

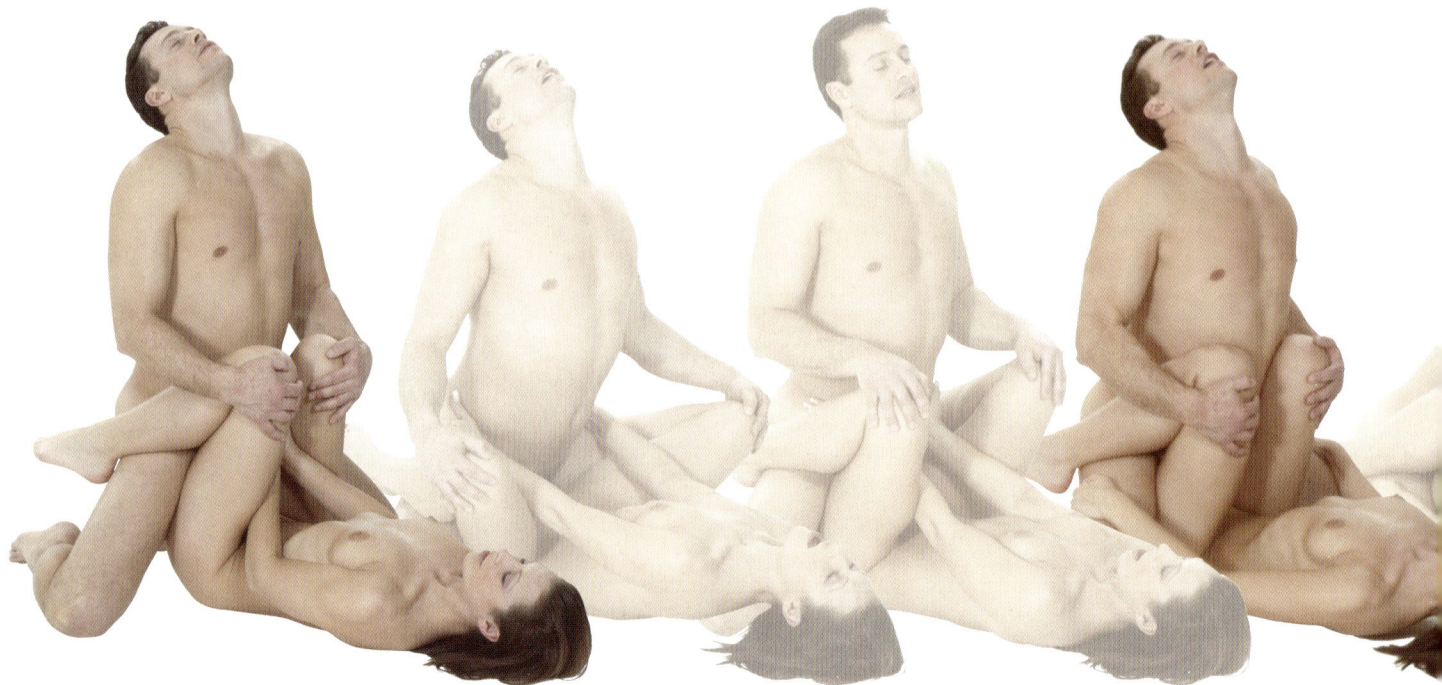

Reliable contraception is a matter for grown-ups, so the book also assumes you have thought this through in advance. So the remaining issues are disappointment, expectation, and frustration, which are best resolved by communication. This means talking to each other openly and honestly.

consent

Before you embark on any sexual experiences and adventures with your partner, you have to make sure that your lover agrees to whatever it is you want to do—and that you are also comfortable with whatever it is they want to do. If you are happy, you can give your consent. This should be spoken out loud so that there are no misunderstandings or any room for misinterpretation of any kind.

We give our consent within whatever boundaries we choose—we will do some things but draw the line at others. Once we have done this, we can use a key word or phrase to stop anything we don't want. It might be as simple as saying "stop." Find out what your lover's boundaries are and under no circumstances ever cross them or put your lover under any pressure to change their parameters; this is unfair. Using emotional blackmail to get your lover to perform a sexual act that they don't want to do is unforgivable. If you value your relationship, don't do it.

Love is more important than sex. Your lover should never be made to feel anything less than your complete and utter heart's desire all the time.

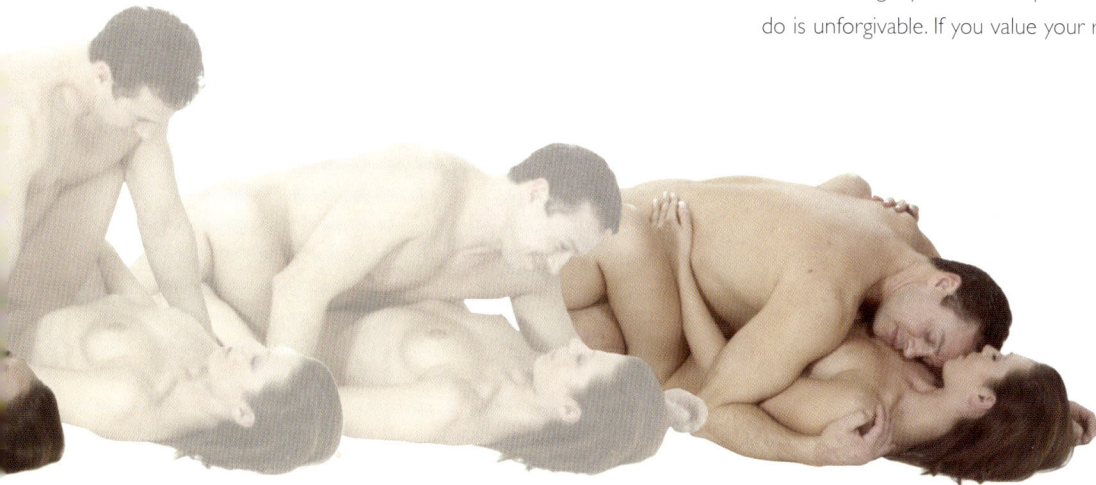

respect

This brings us to our last topic—respect. You have sex with your lover and it is usually implicit that you love them, but you must also like them. Although this sounds obvious, liking them is important. If you don't treat them as well as, if not better than, anyone else you like, then you aren't showing them the proper respect. A lot of couples treat each other appallingly while claiming to love each other and then wonder why the spark disappears and their relationships turns sour. To have a really good sexual relationship, you have to pay a lot of time and attention to respect.

Respect not only means avoiding making your lover to do something they don't want to, it also means giving them the space to be themselves, being more concerned with their satisfaction and enjoyment than with your own, being ready to back off when they want you to, and treating them with kindness, gentleness, and consideration.

aspects of sex

You'd be surprised how many uses people have for sex—and we don't judge. Whatever you use sex for is fine just so long as both you and your partner are in agreement and all the rules of respect are in place. No one should be able to tell you what sex should, or should not, be. Sex is a bit like driving; you can get help to be a better driver, but no one can tell you where you ought to go in your car.

In the West, people tend to think of sex as a quick physical activity, whereas in the East sex has always been seen as a lot more; it is viewed as a serious approach to both spirituality and humanity. While many of the physical positions shown here originated from such works as the famous Indian book, the *Kama Sutra*, do not feel that you must use sex as a spiritual outlet. By all means do so if you wish, but the scope of this book deals mainly with the physical aspects of sex. This means that it shows you how to use your body to improve your lovemaking techniques so you can enjoy sex more on a purely physical level, an enjoyment that will also have a positive effect on your relationship with your lover.

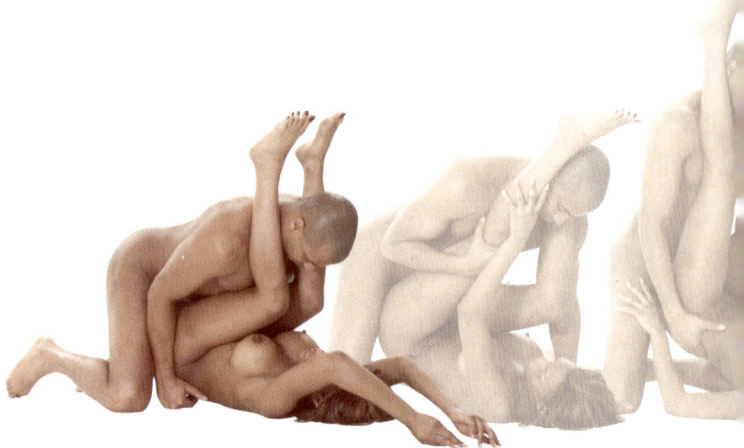

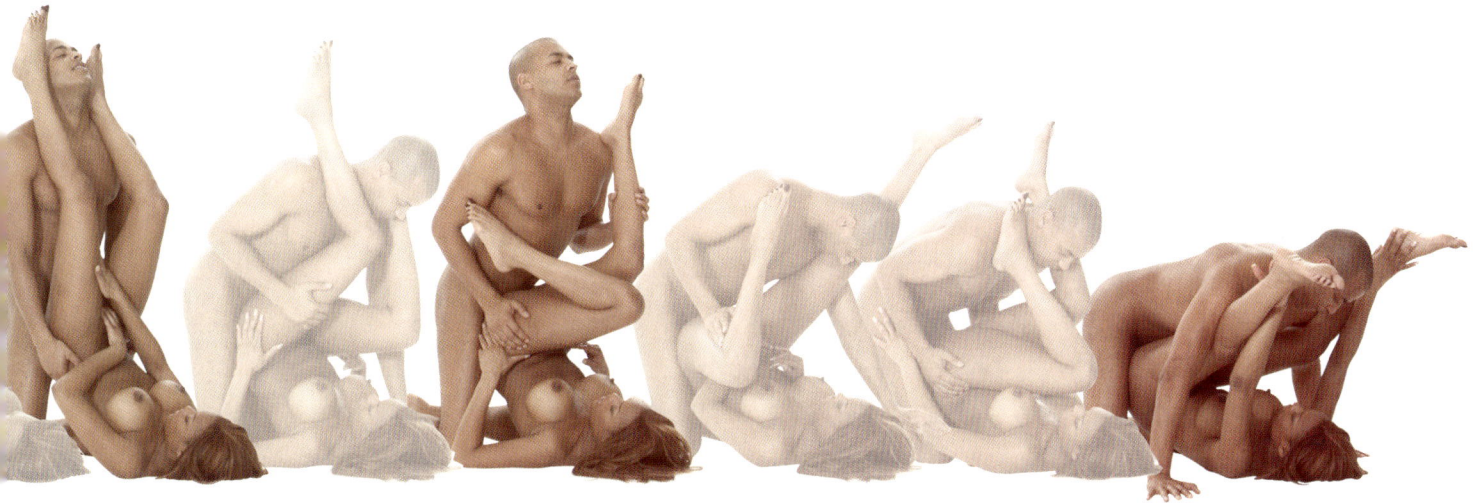

WHAT SORT OF SEX?

There are many different reasons for having sex. You can use it as a tool to:

- express your love for your partner
- meet your own or your partner's needs and desires
- bring a spiritual dimension to your life
- have fun and enjoyment
- exercise your body
- relax
- get to sleep

If you keep practicing and exploring and giving, sex just gets better the longer you are in a relationship. Long-term relationships should produce fantastic sex, but you have to make the effort to keep your imagination working. If you do so, sex should never get boring.

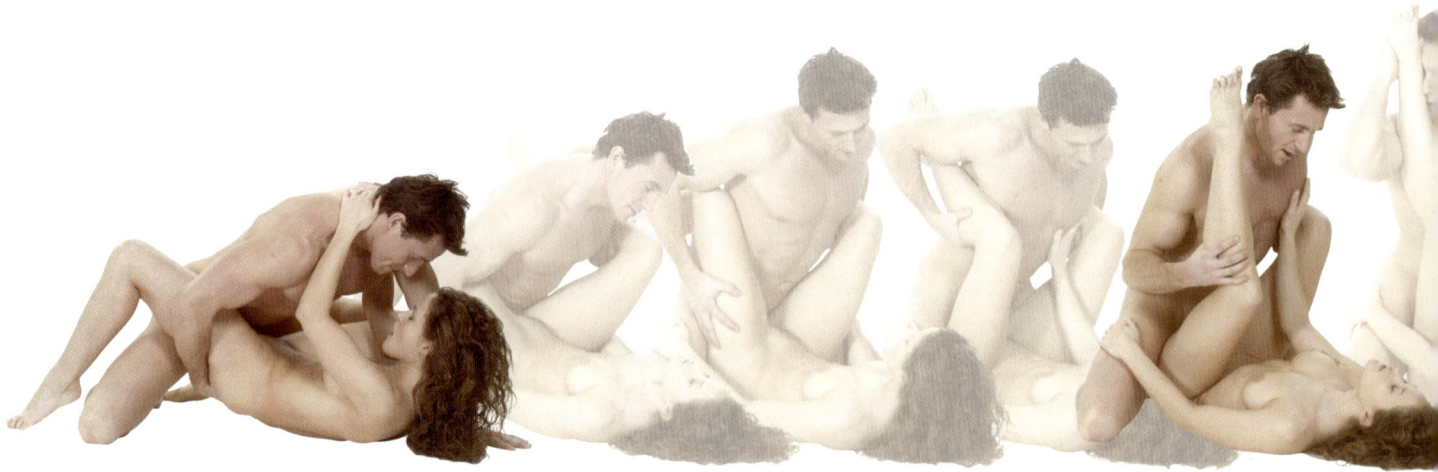

cycles of relationships

There are times when you may not want sex. This can be for a whole variety of reasons—you may be recovering from childbirth or major surgery, or getting over a trauma such as bereavement, redundancy, or nursing a seriously ill child. During these times your libido may drop. A loving partner should accept and understand this and put no pressure on you. But there are times when this low libido can become a long-term problem. If this is the case, consider seeking qualified medical advice.

It is worth bearing in mind that relationships go through quite natural cycles. When we first meet a new lover, our libido is probably at its highest and we can't wait to tear off each other's clothes. The sex during this introductory period is fast and furious, frantic, and frenzied. It's as if we can't get enough of each other—as indeed we can't. Then things quieten a little and we grow closer, more loving. The sex during this secondary period can become almost languid, deeper, more meaningful. Then we enter the third stage when sex may almost disappear completely but the closeness is there, the intimacy. There is an understanding and friendship that may replace the sexual life. If both partners are happy with this, then the relationship continues and is strengthened. If, however, one partner isn't quite ready to forgo sex, then problems may be encountered. As long as

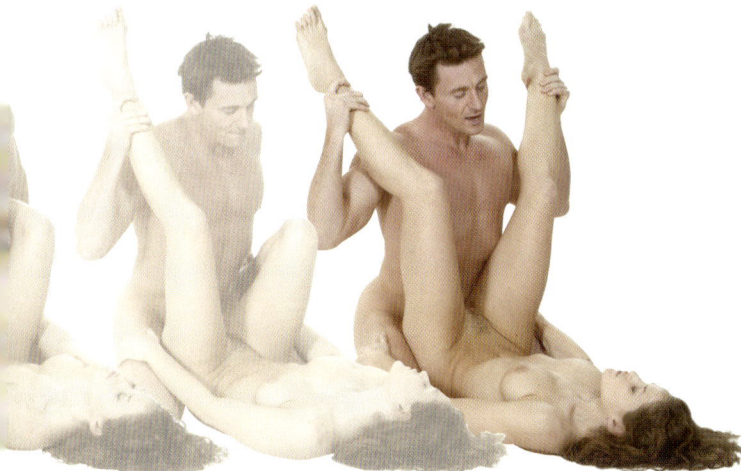

- ■ Don't rush things. Take your time. Turn off phones and pagers.

keeping sex alive

There is a secret kept by many older people—sex just keeps on getting better. Young people think it is all about rush and passion and instant gratification and this can undoubtedly be tremendous fun. But as you get older you may start to want quality over quantity, skill over speed, and long intense orgasms rather than a speedy bout of sex that leaves you both out of breath but feeling unsatisfied.

Sex gets better the more in love you are with your partner. And love gets stronger the more time and emotional energy you put into your relationship. Successful long-term lovers know their way around each other's bodies and know what turns the other on. But they keep experimenting, seducing, teasing, and flirting. The only boring sex is repetitious sex, done by rote, with little or no imagination invested in it. This has nothing to do with age or the length of time you've been in love. Boring sex often starts out that way. Lovers who learn how to experiment often never lose this precious habit.

Nevertheless, we all go through periods when we need less sex than our partner or go off sex altogether. Generally, though, as long as your partner treats you with care and doesn't pressurize you into having sex, your libido will pick up again in time. Caring and loving are the real keys to long-term satisfaction.

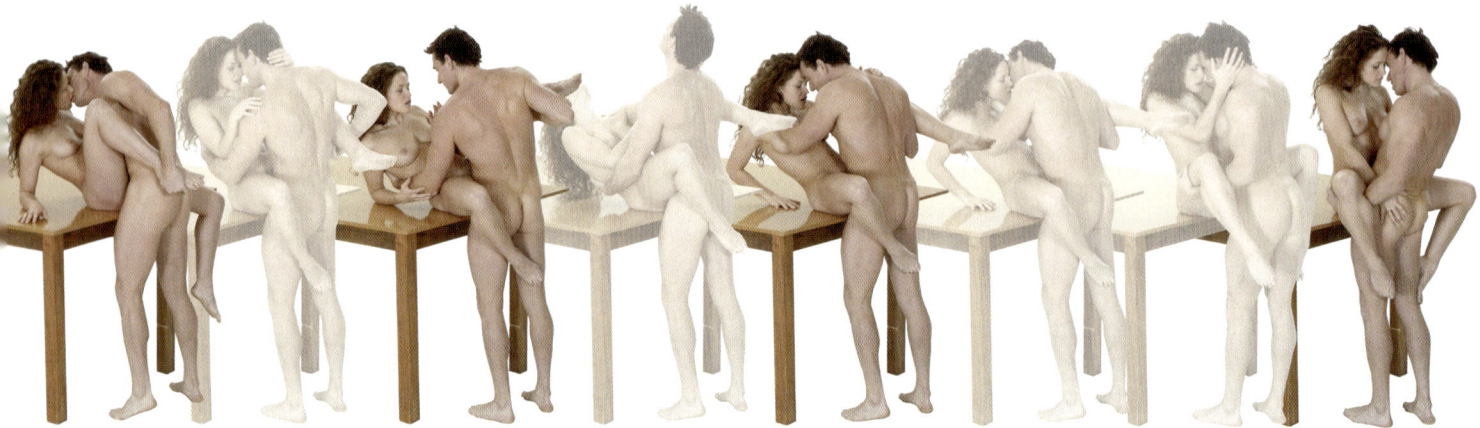

go with the flow

The special Flowmotion images used in this book have been created to show you every stage of the various sexual positions and techniques illustrated, not just selected highlights. The images in each sequence run across the page from left to right and show not only how to perform each technique but also how to get the best out of it, in a detailed and straightforward manner. Each technique or position is fully explained by step-by-step captions. Below this, another layer of information in the timeline breaks the techniques into their various key stages. The symbols in the timeline are instructions for when to move on to the next stage in the sequence, or when to stop before starting the next position.

changing position I | 51

changing position I

Moving from one position to the next should be a smooth operation carried out easily and without having to start again from the beginning. Sometimes neither of you really knows which way to go. Better to tell your partner than to assume and bump into each other going in opposite directions.

● If the woman is astride the man, let her lead the change of position. This way the man does not have to push his partner away. She can simply slide off and pull him onto her ready for the next position.

● It is usually best to say what it is you are doing so that both of you know. That way, there is no scope for misunderstanding. Remember that good communication is good foreplay.

● These movements should be effortless and smooth, but we all make mistakes. Fall over, get it wrong—you can just laugh and have fun. You are changing position, not conducting a business meeting, so enjoy yourselves.

● You might find it more comfortable to do this on or in a bed rather than on a hard floor. As the woman falls backward she brings the man with her and guides him into the next position that she wants to try.

● As the woman lies down, the man has easy access to her and can caress her clitoris and stroke her thighs to further her excitement.

● From this position it is quite easy for the man to maneuver himself, ready for lovemaking in the man-on-top position. Maintain eye contact with each other while doing this to keep the passion going.

● The man then leans forward and kisses his partner. Taking his weight on his arms so that he does not press too hard down on the woman, he is now ready for lovemaking.

● As he enters her, the man should continue to take his weight on his arms. The woman can help him by pulling him closer to her and arching her back to receive him into her.

| ■ | communicate | ▶ | enjoy | ▶ | comfort | ▶ | access | ▶ | maneuver | ▶ | kiss | ▶ | ‖ |

■ This indicates the beginning or end of a sequence.

▶ This indicates continued movement in the sequence.

‖ This indicates a pause between sequences.

foreplay

undressing

Sometimes undressing can be hurried, quick, and urgent, but mostly it will be seductive, slow, erotic, and very sexy. Sometimes you will not even need to get undressed at all. It is worth remembering that keeping a little part of you hidden can be very erotic indeed.

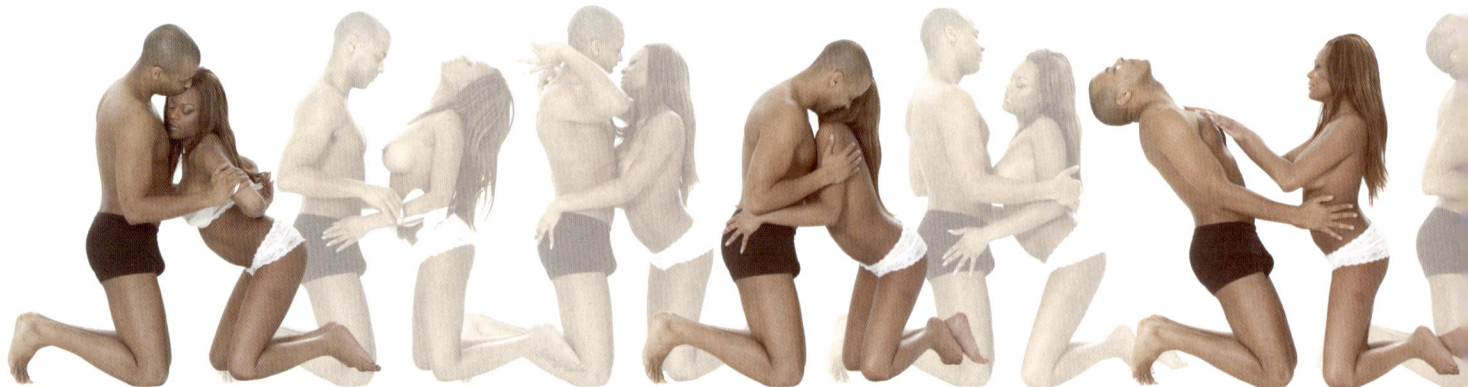

● Whether you undress yourself or let your partner help you out of your clothes, it does not really matter. You can always share the task of fumbling with difficult clasps, zippers, and buttons.

● Being undressed slowly by your lover is a very erotic experience and should not be rushed. Take your time and be sexy—put on a show.

● As you remove each item of clothing, take time to caress the new areas of skin that have been exposed. Resist the urge to hurry the process in the rush to reach total nakedness.

● Foreplay is not something to be rushed. Take time to explore your lover's body using different techniques of caressing and stroking—hard, soft, fun, wet. Enjoy the experience.

be seductive ▶ **don't hurry** ▶ **experiment** ▶

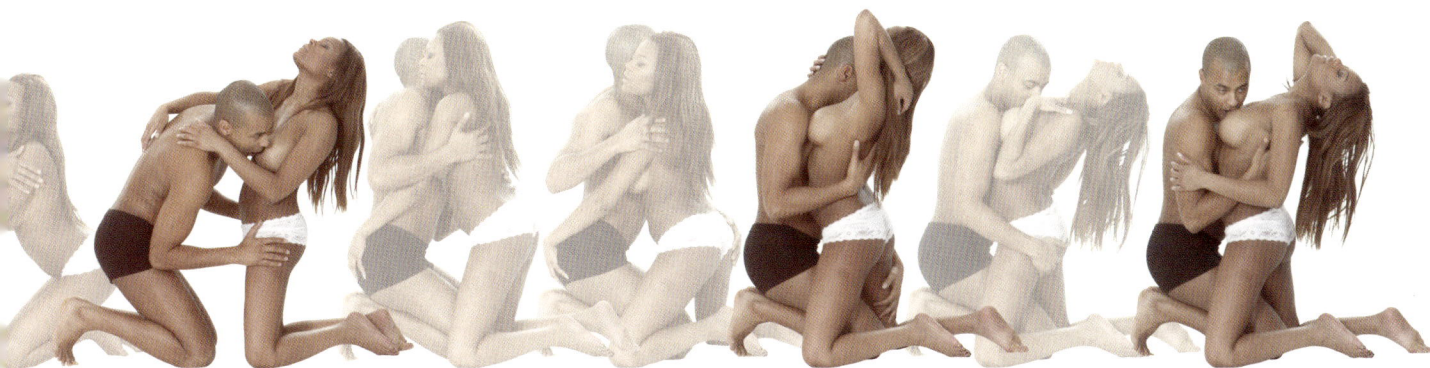

● This is not the time to worry about who makes the next move, orgasms, or satisfaction. Being naked with your lover and enjoying the feel of their skin on yours is enough at the moment.

● Feel the pleasure of just being held by your partner, being wanted, and being made to feel special. This is your lover, so tell them that you love them, kiss them, and be sexy with them.

● Teasing is the essence of foreplay— it gets the juices flowing, so use stroking rather than heavy fondling to excite your partner. The man should also take a gentle approach when handling the woman's breasts.

● While the woman caresses her partner's penis, using subtle touch rather than direct stimulation, the man caresses the woman's nipples to arouse her and make her want more.

enjoy   ►   **get sexy**   ►   **tease**   ►   **II**

embracing

When lovers embrace, they are saying that they love each other through an intimate physical action. There's no need to rush to the next stage of lovemaking. Linger in mutual embrace as long as you wish, enjoying the warmth and the promise of what's to come.

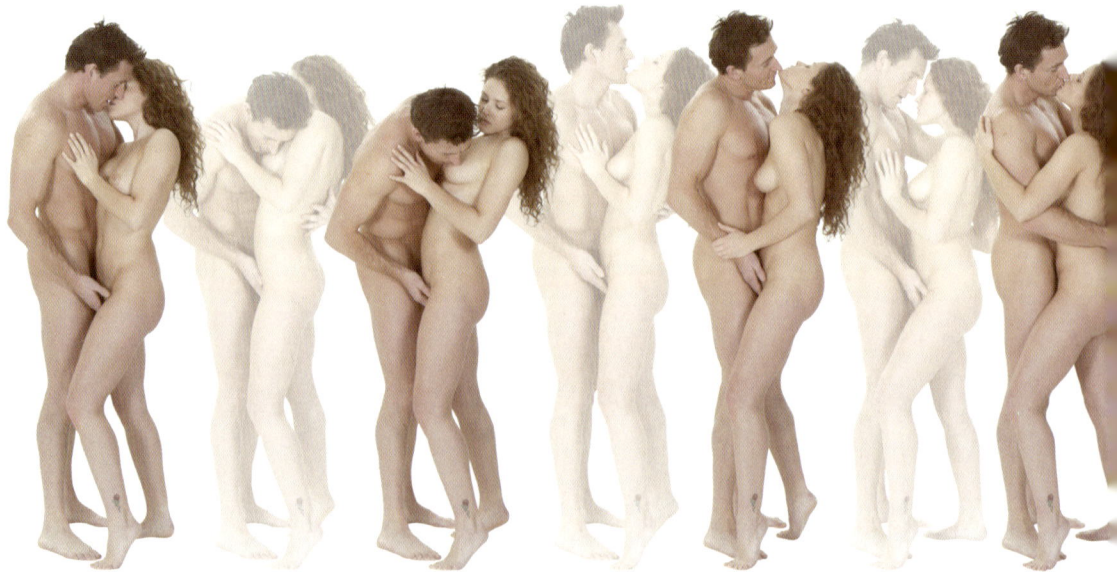

● Sexual excitement can arise at any time but good lovemaking occurs when we feel respected, trusted, accepted, and loved. Prolonged foreplay will enhance the pleasure received and given during sex.

● Embracing is a form of foreplay—it means caressing, stroking, and rubbing your partner gently. Use cuddling and soothing to reassure and to show acceptance. Being naked takes courage and demands your respect and love.

● If you are in a long-term, stable relationship, you will have worked out a series of key words or gestures to convey to your partner when you want them to stop or when you want them to carry on doing something.

● You may, for example, place your hand on your partner's chest to suggest "no," or you may simply say the word. To encourage your partner to continue their actions, try moaning gently or whispering "yes."

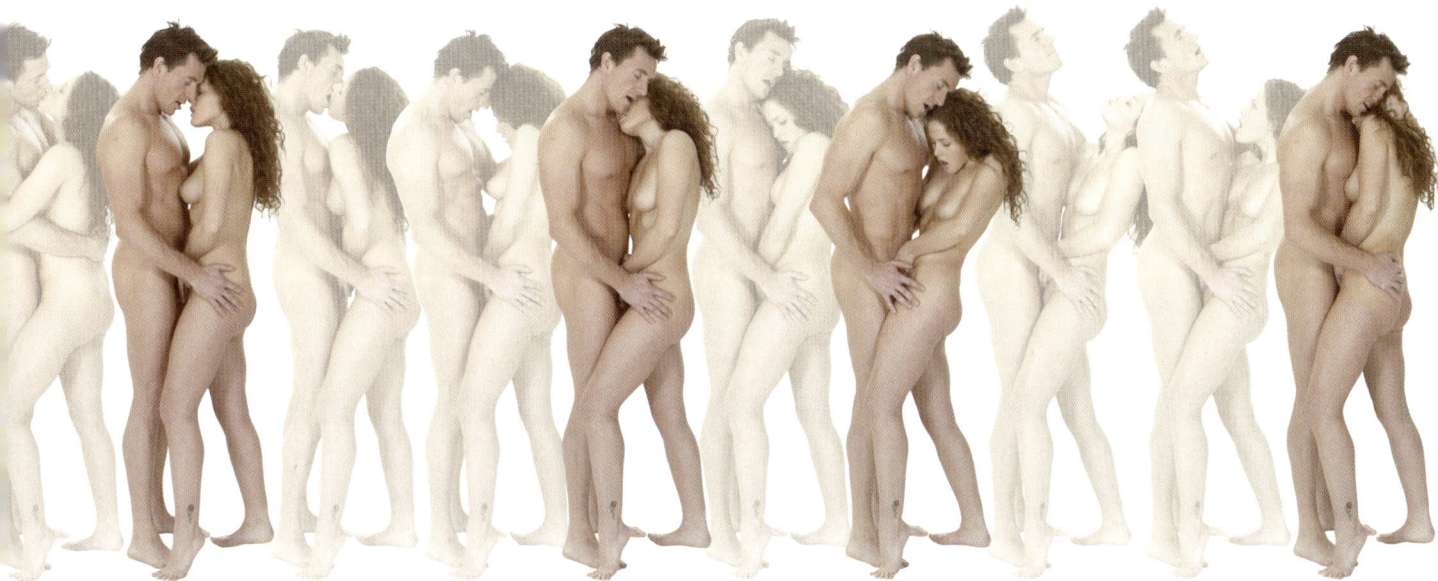

● Have the confidence to explore each other's bodies, experiment and ask for what you want. Remember that being naked also means casting off your emotional inhibitions, so be assertive, be daring.

● Resist trying too hard to make your partner reach orgasm. If it happens that is fine, but foreplay is about teasing, gradually raising the pitch of excitement so that you can move on to other stages of lovemaking.

● When you are being caressed, let yourself lie back and enjoy the attention and sensations. Stop worrying for a moment about your partner's needs and just savor the experience of being loved.

● Try to keep the intimacy going throughout the lovemaking by maintaining eye contact, close hugging, stroking, and being loving. Even when you are in the throes of orgasm, being intimate is rewarding and sexy.

desire ▶ **increase excitement** ▶ **relax** ▶ **II**

masturbation I

For a man, having a woman masturbate him is wonderfully relaxing since it relieves him of all the pressure about performance and prowess. He can simply lie back and enjoy the experience while the woman takes control.

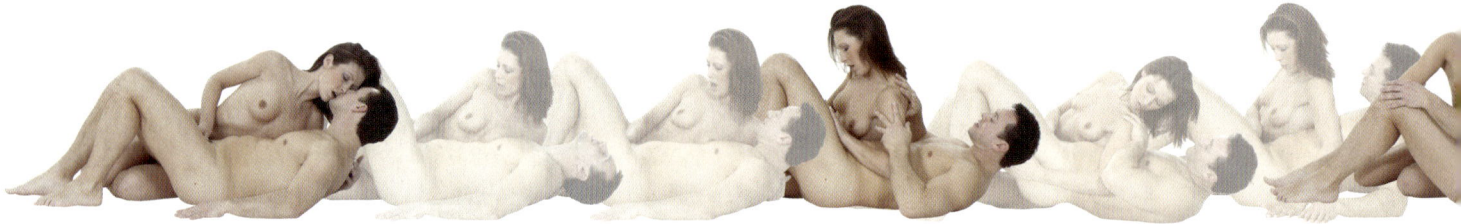

● Lie down together, side by side, and kiss while the woman lightly caresses the man's testicles, thighs, and stomach. Spend time relaxing into the position and resist the urge to rush anything at this stage.

● As she rubs the man's penis, the woman watches his face to gauge his reactions. That way she knows how much pressure to apply.

● Masturbating your lover is more than bringing them to ejaculation. It should be a total experience—visual, emotional, physical, and aural. Admire their body, praise their looks, and tell them how much you love them.

● The woman should try rubbing the penis against her breasts as she masturbates her partner. She can use her nipples to further his stimulation. The man is likely to find this action incredibly sexy.

	enjoy	total experience	be sexy

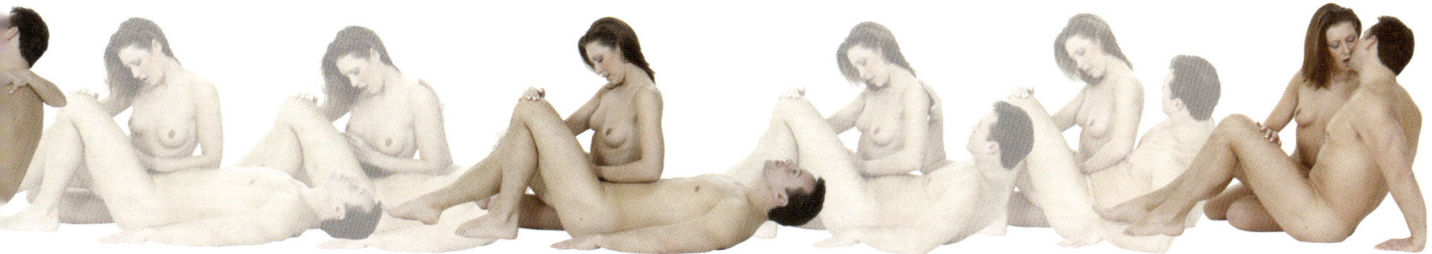

● The woman should use her free hand to keep up a continual caress. She can even masturbate herself to increase further the visual experience for her partner.

● As the man ejaculates, the woman increases his pleasure by varying the intensity and pressure of her hand movements. You will learn with experience what works best for your partner at this stage.

● Some couples find it quite sexy when the man ejaculates over the woman. To achieve this, the woman aims her partner's penis to come over her stomach or breasts.

● As his orgasm subsides, the couple finish off with a kiss and cuddle. If they want to enjoy more lovemaking, the woman continues to handle the penis to stop it getting too soft.

masturbation II

Not all sex has to be of the full-on sort. Sometimes a little light masturbation is all that is needed when we are tired or stressed or if the woman is heavily pregnant. The initial stages of masturbation are always a good part of foreplay anyway, enhancing excitement and stimulation.

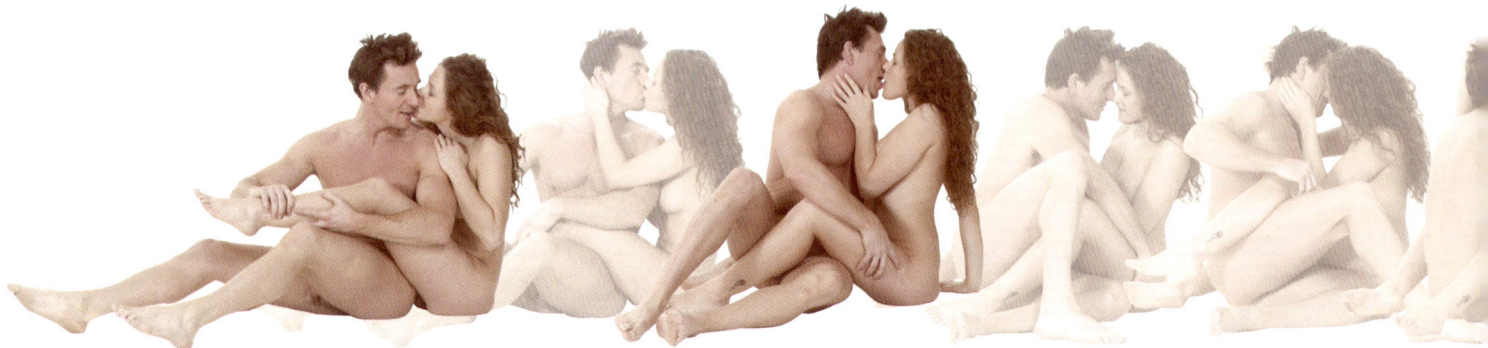

● With the woman sitting behind the man, she reaches forward to stimulate his penis with her hands. Alternatively, the man can masturbate himself while his partner watches.

● The woman gradually moves herself into a position facing the man, from where he will be able to stimulate her clitoris. Keep kissing and maintain close intimate contact with each other all the way through.

● The man then guides the woman's legs over his so that she is nestled in his lap. He strokes her thighs and the woman grasps his penis tightly.

● The couple kiss passionately as the man pushes her legs apart to gain access to her. He can now begin to stimulate her clitoris.

■ **be intimate** ▶ **stroke** ▶ **be passionate** ▶

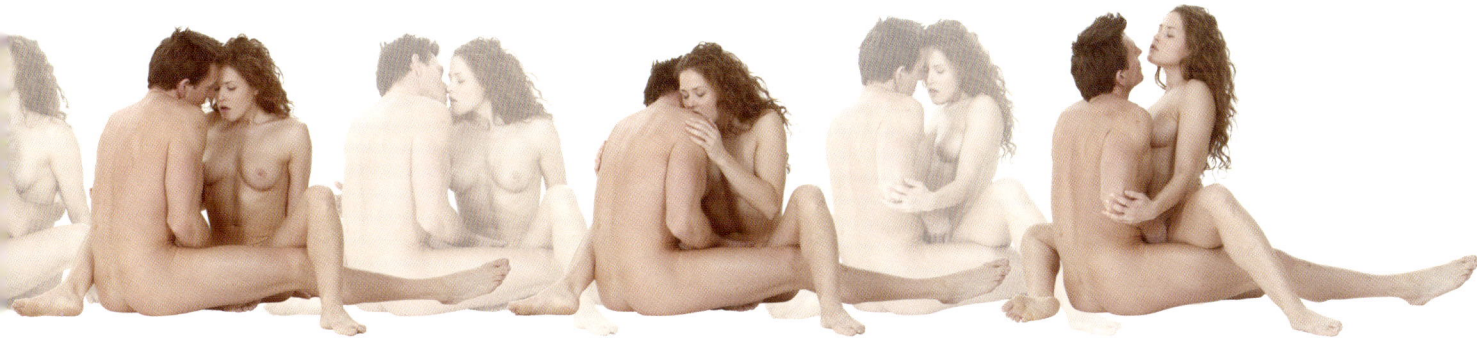

● As the couple sit facing each other they both have access to his penis and her clitoris. He can masturbate himself while she watches or he can masturbate her.

● This is a fun, raunchy position as either of you can masturbate the other. Remember to maintain eye contact and kiss each other for maximum sensation and enjoyment.

● If the woman forces her legs as wide as possible, the man can mount his fingers as he rubs her clitoris faster and harder. If the timing is good, he will be able to masturbate both of them so that they orgasm together.

● As the woman climaxes, she might like to take over from her partner so that he can masturbate himself and ejaculate onto her as he reaches his own orgasm.

kiss ▶   orgasm ▶   II

oral sex I

For some, oral sex is a forerunner to full sex, while for others it is an experience in its own right. It can also be both at different times. Good oral sex requires the man to be part gymnast and part contortionist, but always a very caring man. The woman has to trust her partner completely for her to be so intimate.

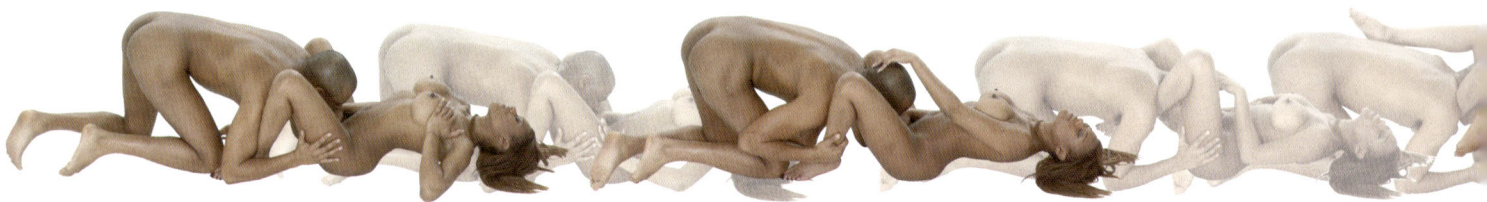

● The woman lies down and lets her raised knees relax out to the sides. In a kneeling position, the man leans forward between the woman's knees and caresses her thighs.

● The man uses his tongue, fingers, lips, and hands to stimulate his partner. The woman is likely to experience greater sensation if he runs his tongue up and around the sides of the clitoris rather than stimulating it directly.

● To give the man better access to her, the woman arches her back. She can gently push his head down, tell him directly, and use moans and sighs to let her partner know that the pressure and rhythm is right.

● The man uses his tongue and lips on the woman's clitoris. Once her vagina is moist, he gently inserts one finger to stimulate her G spot. He can also place his finger in her anus and use his thumb inside her vagina.

stimulate indirectly ▶ **give encouragement** ▶ **be dexterous** ▶

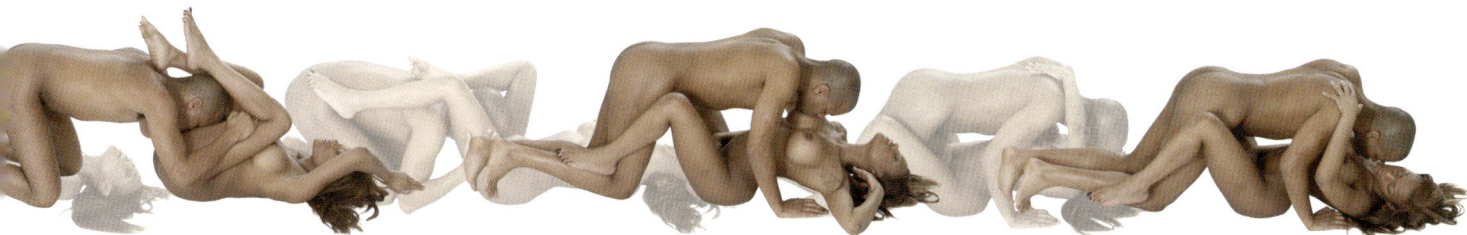

● As the woman's excitement rises, her nipples become erect, her breathing is shallower and faster, and her face becomes flushed. These signs tell her partner that it is time to turn up the tempo of rhythm and pressure.

● Nearing orgasm, the woman may thrash around and become vocal. The man can place more pressure on the clitoris and move his tongue more rapidly to help, but he needs to pace himself so as not to tire too soon.

● As the woman reaches orgasm, her feelings may become so intense that she pushes the man's head or hand away. The man should respect this and realize that his partner does not want to be touched.

● If the woman wants the man to enter her as or just after she climaxes he can quickly slide up her body and enter her to make love.

increase tempo　▶　　　**orgasm**　▶　　　**‖**

oral sex II

There are various positions for a woman to give her man oral sex. Him sitting astride her is one of the easiest, just so long as he can reach orgasm in this kneeling position.

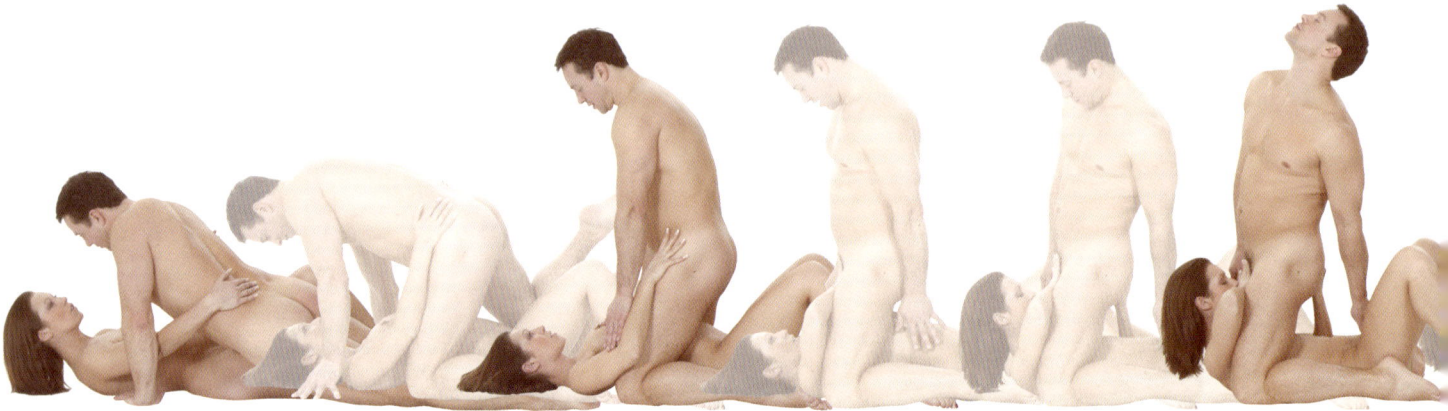

● Lie together with the woman on her back, and embrace. The man gradually eases his way up his partner's body until he is kneeling astride her chest. This position allows her to reach his penis comfortably.

● As the man straddles his partner and moves toward her chest, the woman guides his penis to be cradled in the valley of her breasts. The man is likely to find this act of stimulation incredibly sexy.

● Once the man is kneeling upright, the woman strokes his penis and testicles before taking him into her mouth to suck him. If it is painful for the penis to be pulled downward, she can lift her head to give full oral sex.

● During oral sex, the man should avoid thrusting too hard so as not to cause the woman to gag. She can regulate his thrust by placing one hand on his stomach to push him back.

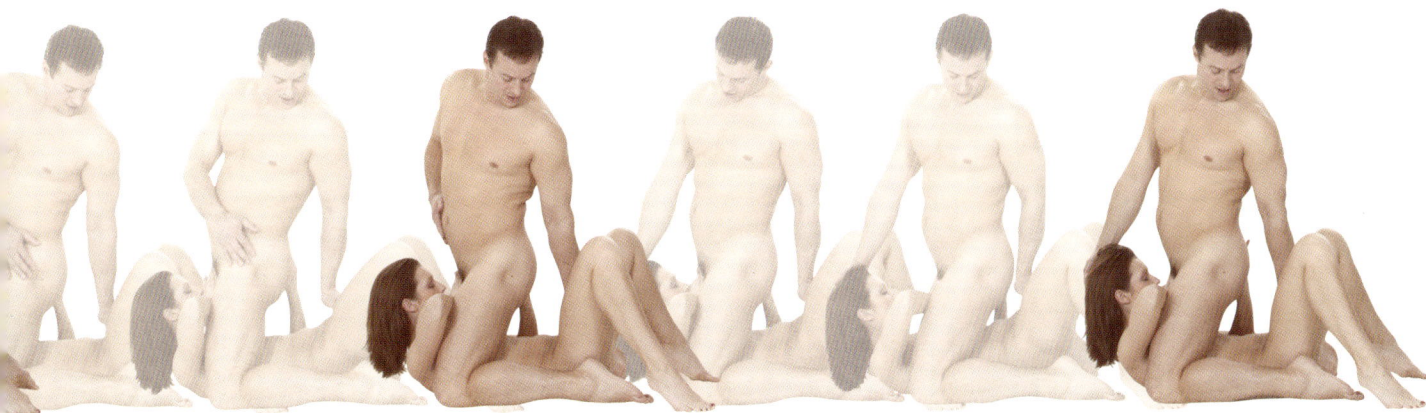

● To help her partner reach orgasm, the woman fondles his buttocks and can insert one finger into his anus for extra stimulation. By twisting slightly, the man can reach her vagina and stimulate her clitoris with his fingers.

● He also strokes and caresses her breasts, or supports her head with his hand. As the woman sucks the penis, she can also masturbate the man by making a fist around his penis or by using the tips of her fingers.

● If the woman does not want her partner to orgasm in her mouth, she should be ready to pull the penis out as he climaxes and let the man ejaculate on her face or breasts.

● Once the man has come he may want to carry on stimulating the woman so that she too can reach orgasm, or he may want to slide off and rest for a moment.

use extra stimulation ▶ **caress** ▶ **orgasm** ▶ II

oral sex III

Oral sex can be enjoyed in all sorts of positions and at many different times during lovemaking. From this standing position, either the man or the woman can be the recipient. Decide which of you is going to pleasure the other and then follow the suggestions below.

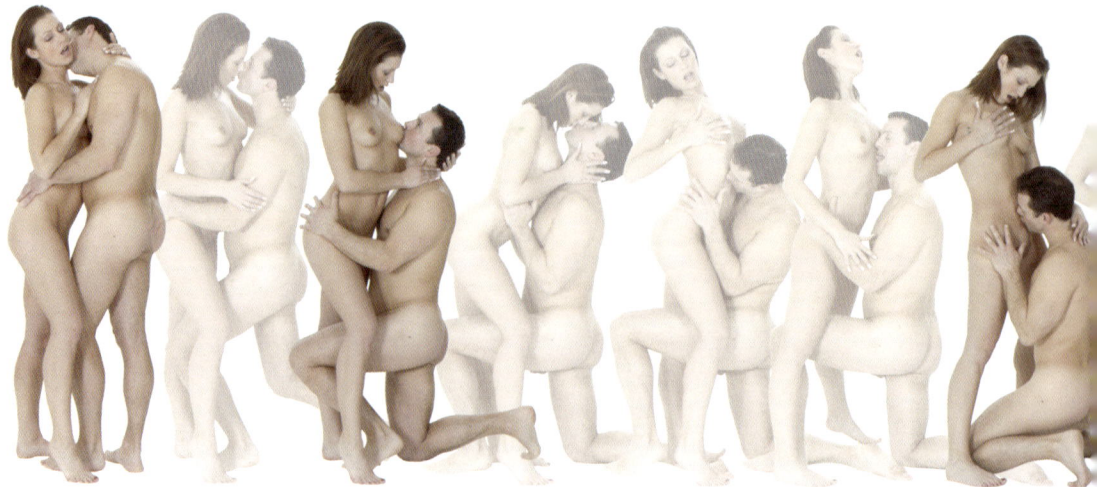

● Good foreplay includes lots of kissing. Kissing means lots of tongue play and lots of caressing and stroking. Nothing feels as good as bare skin and your lover's hands.

● Yes, kissing means mouths, but there is no part of your lover's body that should not be kissed—and stroked, caressed, touched, licked, and sucked.

● If the man is going to pleasure his partner with oral sex, it is best if he takes his time, teasing and arousing her before he actually starts to kiss and lick her clitoris.

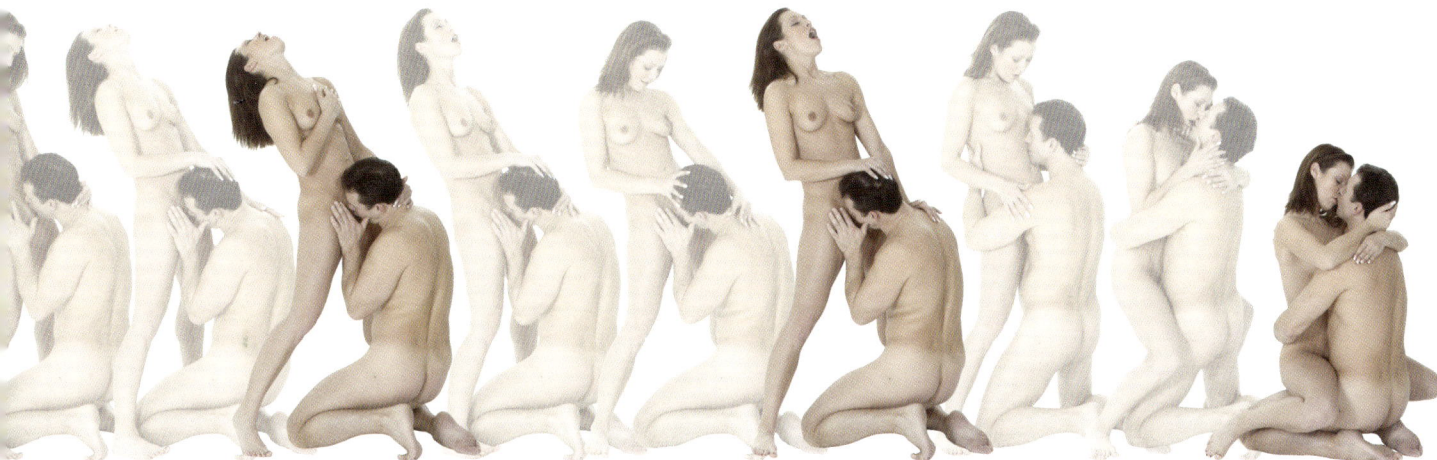

● While the man licks her clitoris, the woman thrusts hard against him. He can also use his fingers to increase her excitement. Seeing your partner kneeling at your feet and taking you in their mouth is a very erotic sight.

● As the woman reaches orgasm, she may press her partner's head harder into her groin and thrust against him. The man can use one hand to hold hard against her buttocks and pull her toward him.

● As her orgasm subsides, the woman may not want to be touched intimately. The man may find that she prefers to be held affectionately, gently, and lovingly in an embrace.

● Gradually the woman slides down the man's body until she is sitting astride his lap. From this position, he can enter her after her orgasm and continue making love to her.

excite   ▶   **orgasm**   ▶   **embrace**   ▶

69 foreplay

Having sex should be fun. You do not have to be all serious. Try lots of things and, above all, remember to enjoy the journey and not worry about the destination. Sometimes it is really satisfying to try lots of different positions first, then end up in the classic 69 and orgasm together.

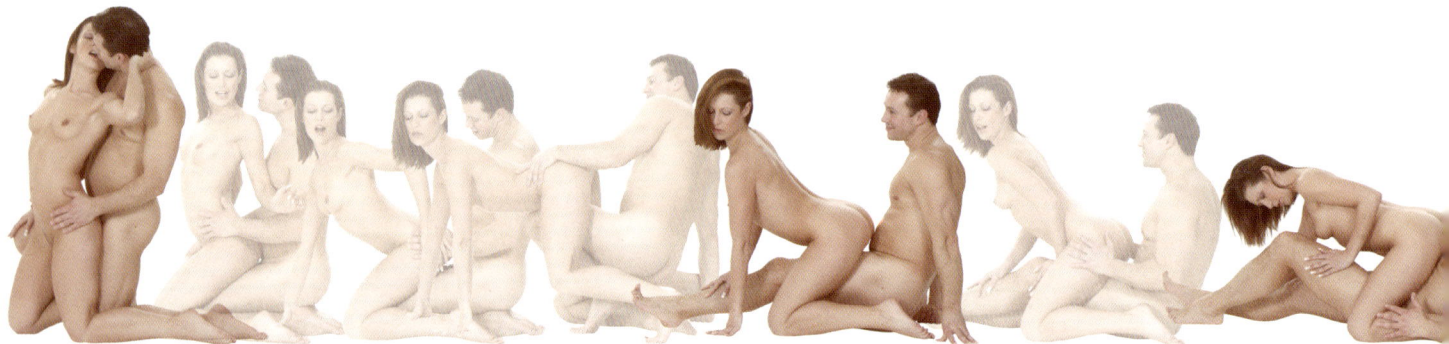

● Once you shed the goal-driven focus, sex becomes much more enjoyable. Freed from any worry about performance or achievements, you are able to concentrate on enjoying and sharing pleasures.

● Still caressing and embracing each other, gradually move into a position where the woman is astride the man with her back facing toward him. This position allows the man to enter her from behind.

● Traditionally, 69 was always called the fantasy position because neither lover can see the other, so they can each fantasize that they are having sex with someone else—this is harmless and fun.

● The woman gradually lowers her body forward, allowing the man a good view of her buttocks which he caresses gently.

■　　　　　　　　**move gradually**　▶　　　**live a fantasy**　▶　　　**caress**　　　　▶

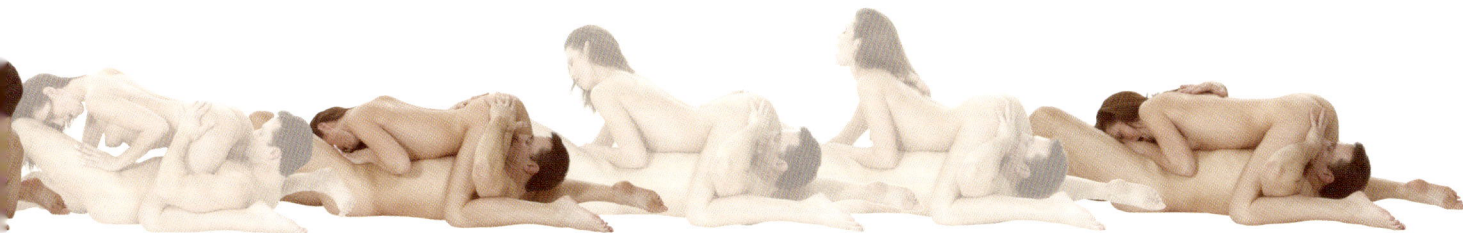

● As she slides down on his body, the woman presents her vagina to her partner for oral sex. At the same time she reaches forward to hold the man's penis in her hand, and then takes him in her mouth.

● If intercourse has taken place before moving into this position, the woman can taste her own juices. Many men find this action very erotic, but it is entirely up to the woman whether she does this.

● Good communication is needed if you want to come simultaneously. Let your partner know how close you are to orgasm so that they can slow down or speed up to keep apace.

● You may not be able to concentrate quite so well on your own orgasm or, if you do, you may lose contact with your partner's climax. Remember that sometimes giving pleasure can be better than receiving it.

69 II *foreplay*

Enjoying oral sex at the same time as your partner is slightly more involved than when just one of you is the recipient. It can also be quite difficult for both of you to orgasm simultaneously. But it is still very stimulating and worth the effort if only to enjoy each other's pleasure.

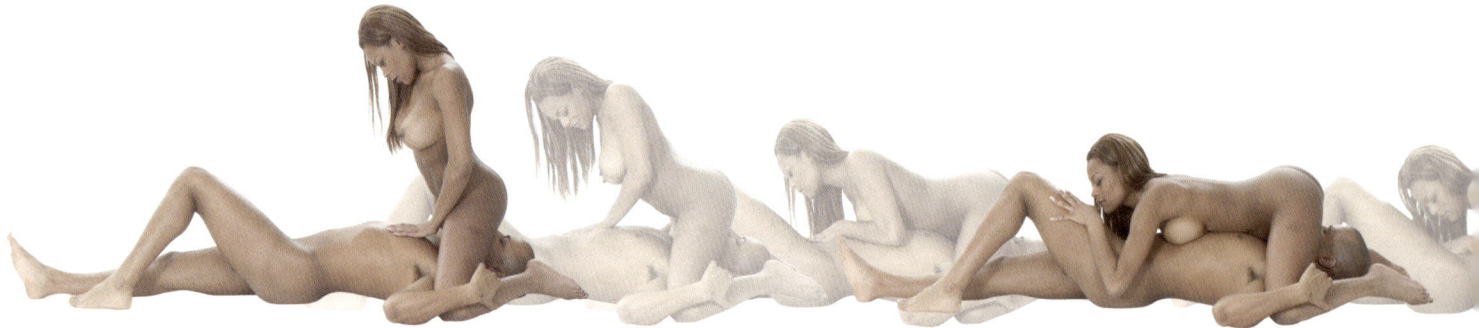

● The best way to start is for the man to lie down and the woman to kneel astride his face. This gives him clear access to her vagina and he can start to lick and suck her clitoris.

● As the man stimulates her clitoris, the woman slowly slides down his body, licking his nipples as she goes and rubbing his chest and stomach.

● When she reaches his penis, the woman delays slightly from taking him in her mouth to tease him. Rub his penis and stroke him sexily but make him wait just a little longer before you start oral sex.

● The woman should take a moment to pause and enjoy the oral sex being performed on her. Experience the sensual touch of your partner's tongue and their fingers caressing your body.

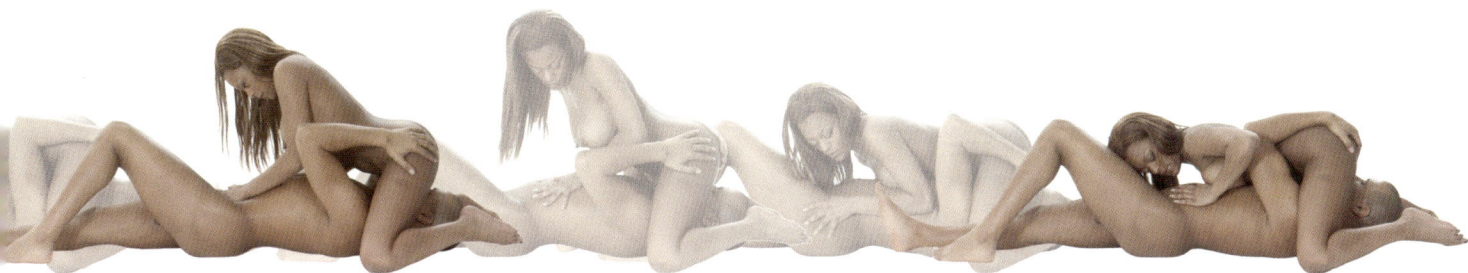

● Take a break from oral sex at any time to get your breath back. Just remember to continue stroking and to maintain the physical contact while you pause, so as to keep the levels of passion at a high pitch.

● If the woman is close to orgasm, she should feel free to come. Mutual oral sex does not have to be goal-driven to be exciting. Enjoy your own orgasm, knowing that you will help your partner come in due course.

● Few men are able to reach orgasm by being sucked only, so the woman needs to masturbate the penis with her hand at the same time. Good oral sex is a matter of combined rhythm—sucking with masturbation.

● It is entirely up to the woman whether she lets the man come in her mouth and, if she does, whether she swallows or not. Do not ever make her do anything she does not feel entirely comfortable with.

relax ‖ ▶ **be considerate** ▶ **rhythm** ▶ ‖

having fun

Lovemaking and foreplay do not have to be all serious and intense. You are allowed to have fun, to laugh, and to let your hair down. Let yourself be wild, silly, athletic, daring, and adventurous.

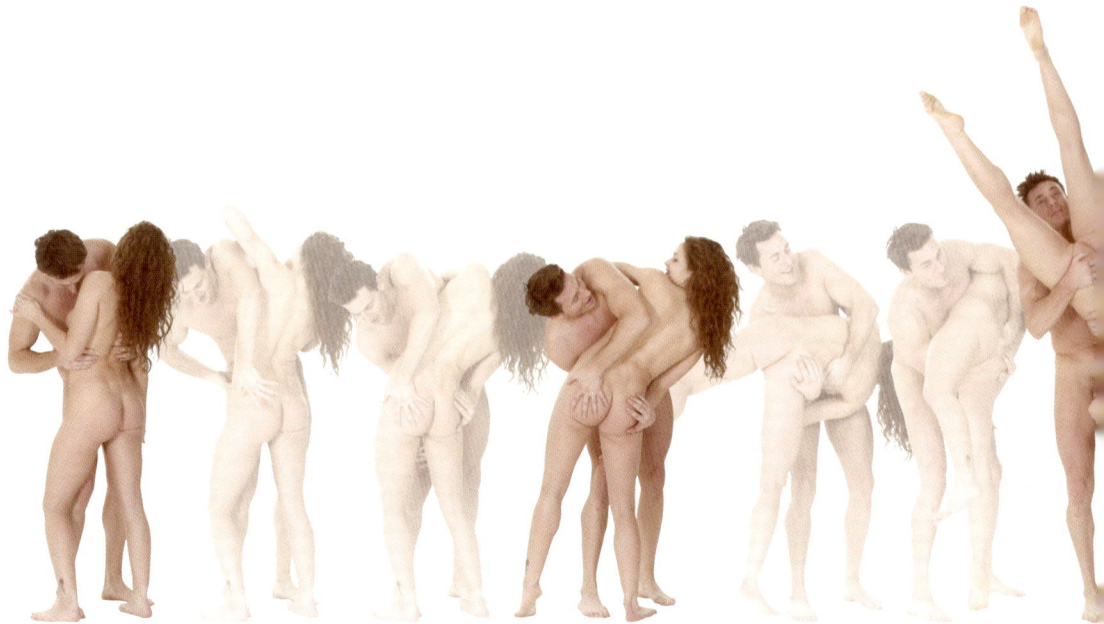

● You both have to be fairly fit and athletic to try this. If you are not, it does not matter—having fun is the name of the game—but do not attempt it if either of you suffers from serious back problems.

● Stand facing each other in an embrace. As the man grasps his partner by the buttocks, the woman should grip him around the lower back. Keep the movements gentle to avoid knocking each other off balance.

● As the man swings the woman upside down, she slides down his back and grasps his thighs firmly. The man can then hold his partner around the waist and buttocks.

■ have fun   1-2-3 go   ▶   grip firmly   ▶

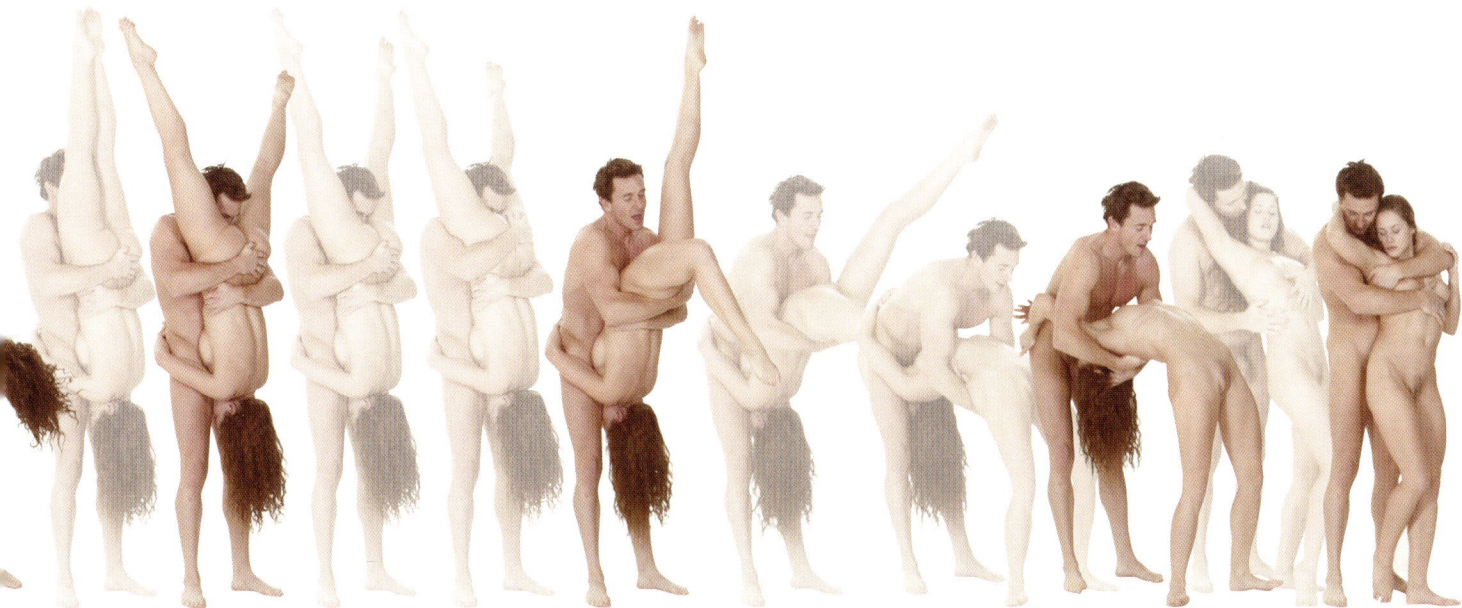

● Once the woman is upside-down, she parts her legs to give the man oral access to her. At the same time, she is able to take her partner in her mouth—this is 69 for the seriously fit.

● Unless you are confident that you have the stamina, it is probably best if neither of you orgasms in this position, to avoid the danger of relaxing your hold on each other. Make sure you do not lose your balance and fall over.

● From this position the man gently lowers the woman forward, supporting her back until her feet are firmly on the floor.

● Once the woman is in the standing position, either with her back to her partner or facing him, the couple can caress and kiss. Alternatively, the woman could bend forward ready for the man to enter her from behind.

getting ready

foreplay

This is the point when all the pleasures, build-up, intimacy, warmth, and anticipation of foreplay come to a natural end and your real lovemaking begins.

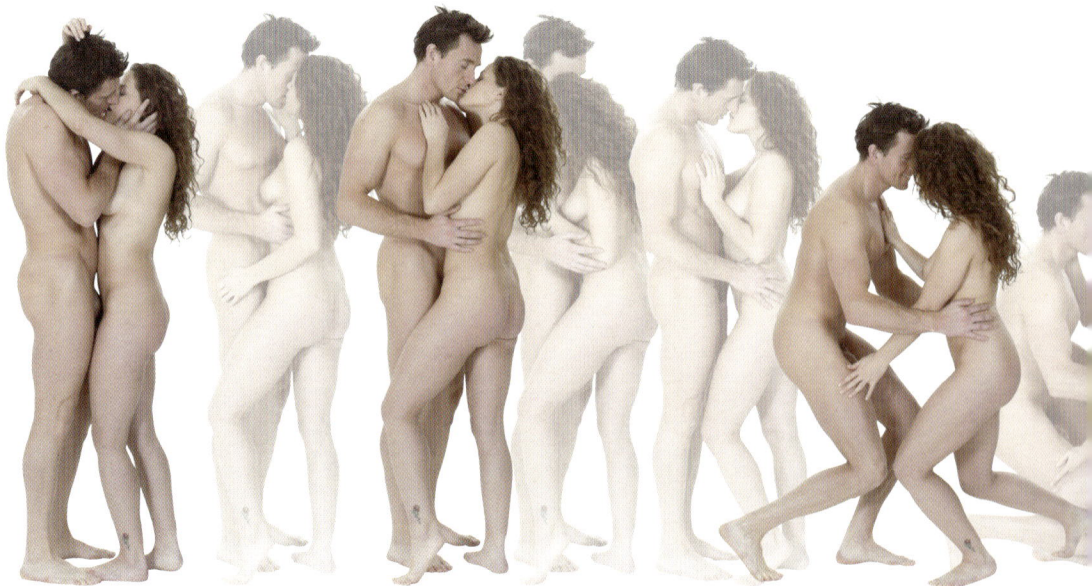

● If you are both standing up and fall onto a bed to make love, it is a lot easier than falling to the ground in the heat of passion. You want to make this transition as easily as possible without embarrassment or awkwardness.

● When you reach the time for lovemaking, one of you should take the lead. Still embracing each other, let one partner gently guide the other in the descent to the floor. This move should be practiced and smooth.

● As you slide down your partner's body, remember to keep caressing and kissing. Use gestures to pull your partner slowly down with you.

● Each take a step back to give yourselves room to maneuver into the kneeling position. Continue to face each other, remembering to maintain eye contact and touch.

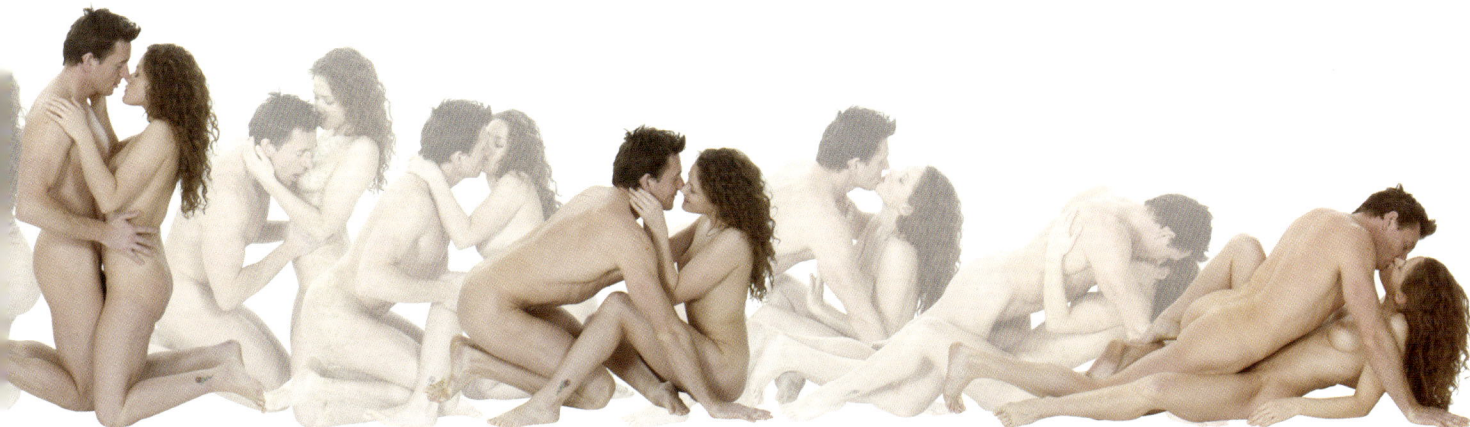

● Once you are both in the kneeling position, the man leans forward to kiss the woman's breasts while she pulls him tightly to her body.

● You will now find it quite easy to slide downward onto the floor ready to begin making love. One of you should be leading, the other following.

● As the woman lowers herself onto her back, the man uses his arms to support his body weight as he follows her lead. Once she is lying on her back, the woman is ready to receive her partner on top of her.

● When you are both ready to have sex, the woman spreads her legs wide to allow her partner to maneuver himself between her legs and prepare to enter her.

be loving ▶ **lead** ▶ **lie down** ▶ ‖

changing position I

Moving from one position to the next should be a smooth operation carried out easily and without having to start again from the beginning. Sometimes neither of you really knows which way to go. It's better to tell your partner than to assume and bump into each other going in opposite directions.

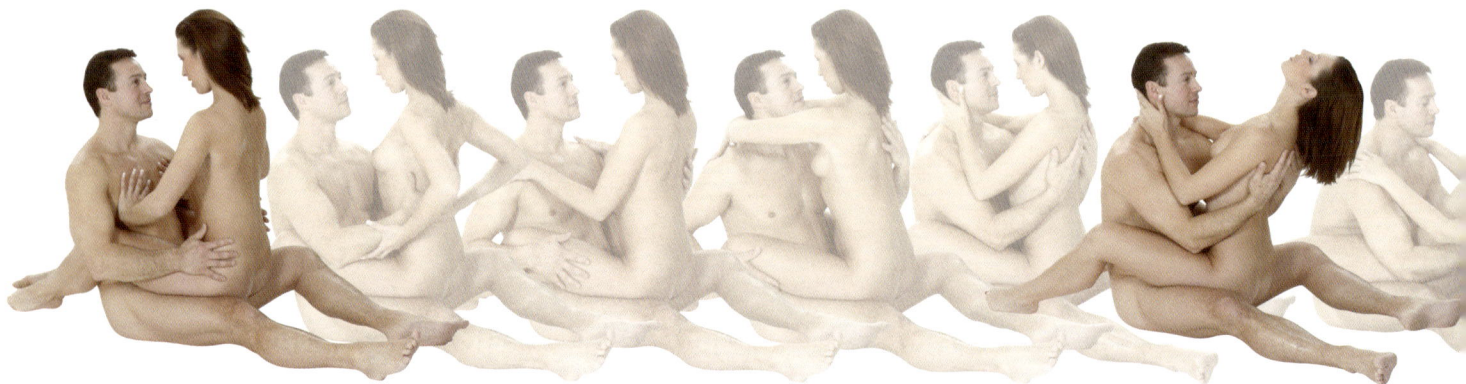

● If the woman is astride the man, let her lead the change of position. This way the man does not have to push his partner away. She can simply slide off and pull him onto her ready for the next position.

● It is usually best to say what it is you are doing so that both of you know. That way, there is no scope for misunderstanding. Remember that good communication is good sex.

● These movements should be effortless and smooth, but we all make mistakes. Fall over, get it wrong—you can just laugh and have fun. You are changing position, not conducting a business meeting, so enjoy yourselves.

● You might find it more comfortable to do this on or in a bed rather than on a hard floor. As the woman falls backward, she brings the man with her and guides him into the next position that she wants to try.

communicate ▶ enjoy ▶ comfort ▶

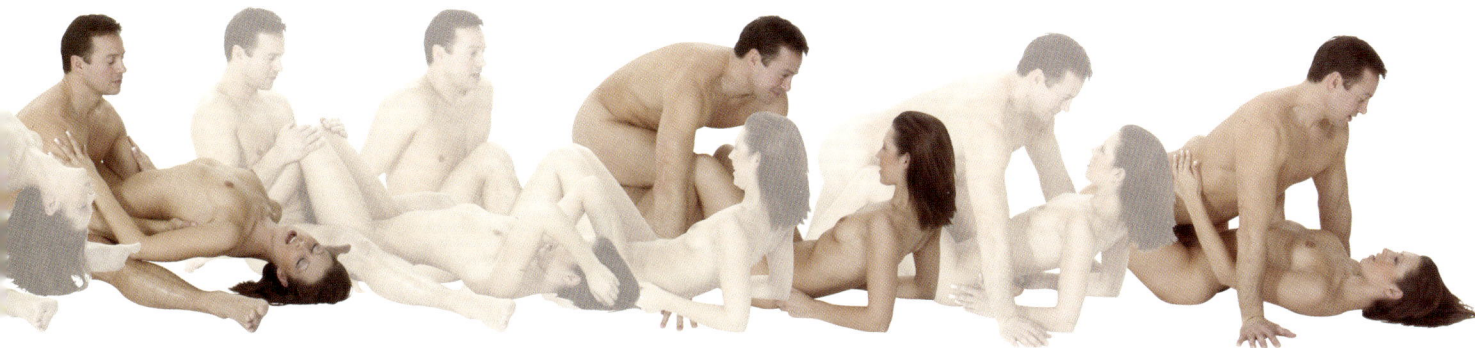

● As the woman lies down, the man has easy access to her and can caress her clitoris and stroke her thighs to further her excitement.

● From this position it is quite easy for the man to maneuver himself, ready for lovemaking in the man-on-top position. Maintain eye contact with each other while doing this to keep the passion going.

● The man then leans forward and kisses his partner. Taking his weight on his arms so that he does not press down too hard on the woman, he is now ready for lovemaking.

● As he enters her, the man should continue to take his weight on his arms. The woman can help him by pulling him closer to her and arching her back to receive him into her.

access ▶ **maneuver** ▶ **kiss** ▶ II

foreplay

changing position II

If the woman is stimulating the man with oral sex and then wants him to enter her, she can slide effortlessly up his body and sit astride him easily.

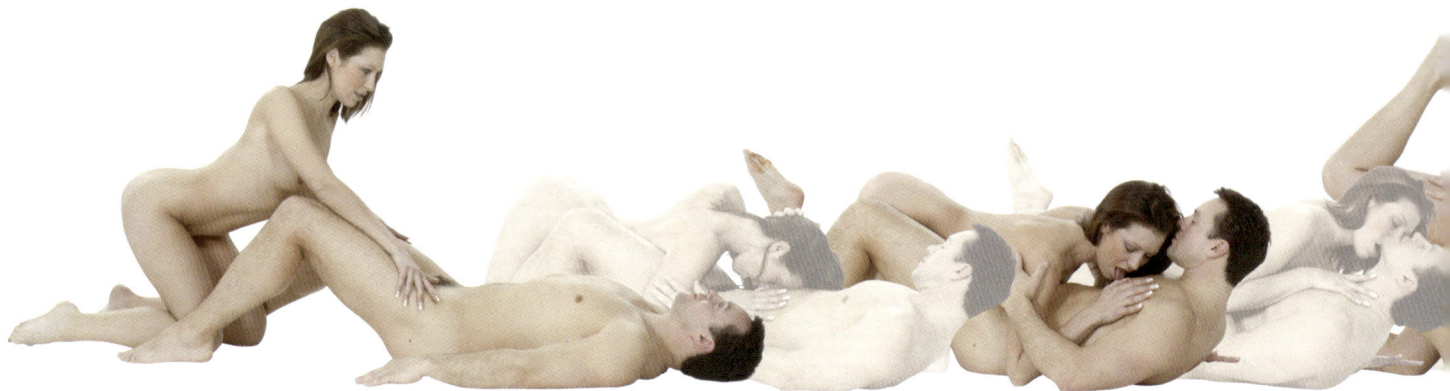

● With the man lying down in a relaxed position, the woman should gently caress her partner's thighs and excite him until he is ready for oral sex. She can then masturbate his penis with her hands.

● As the woman takes the man into her mouth, she continues to caress him with her hands. One hand can caress his testicles while the other hand could stimulate his perineum or lightly play with his nipples.

● By letting her breasts and erect nipples lightly brush across the man's knees, the woman increases the stimulation for her partner.

● As the man's excitement increases, but before he ejaculates, the woman gently slides up her partner's body. If she has a moist vagina, the sensation of her wetness against his skin will be a very thrilling experience.

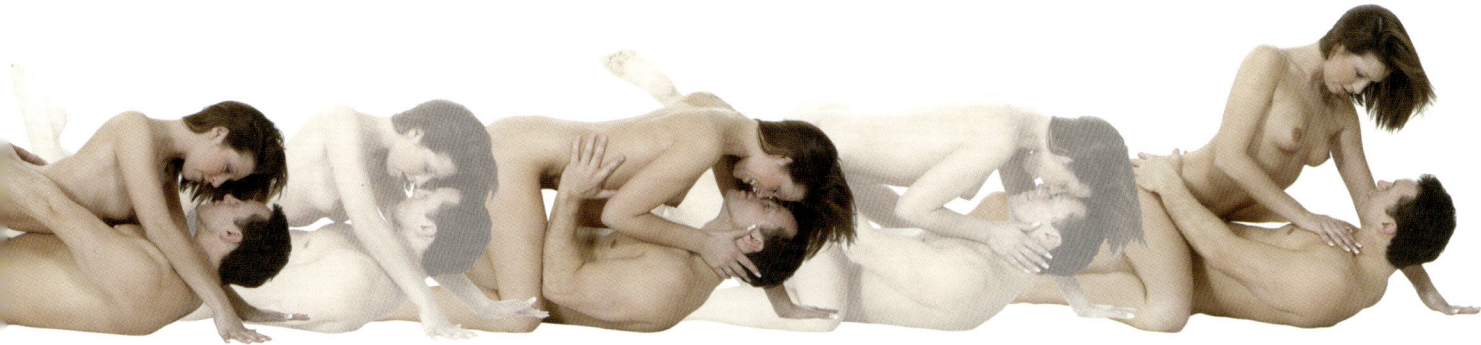

● To further his excitement, the woman presses her pubic region hard against the man's erect penis, helped by him clasping her buttocks. Give each other a hard kiss as you meet face to face.

● As the woman begins to mount her partner, she leans forward to let him caress her breasts and suck her nipples. He can run his hands down her body and along her buttocks and then stimulate her clitoris.

● Keeping one hand on the floor for support, the woman gradually raises herself into the sitting position, astride the man. Kneeling across his thighs, she can still lean forward to carry on kissing and caressing him.

● Once she is fully upright, the woman slides her knees forward. The man enters her, holding her body against his. Using her knees, the woman levers herself up and down to help her partner reach climax easily.

standing positions

grapevine I

Most of the standing positions for lovemaking require a certain degree of fitness and strength. You may not achieve full satisfaction from it, but you will certainly have fun trying.

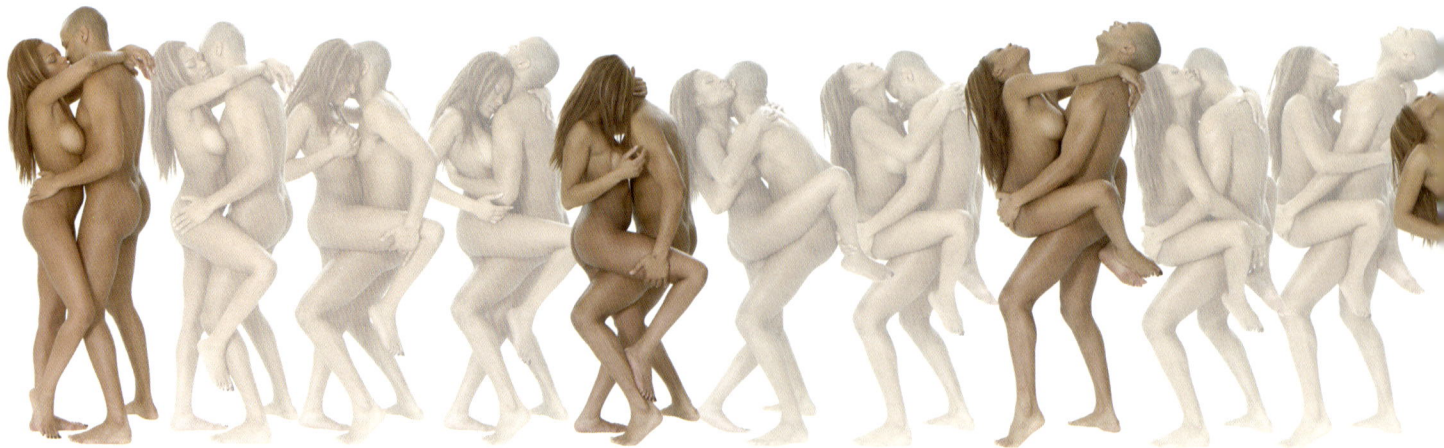

● If the couple stand face to face, they can caress each other and kiss. The woman places her arms around the man's neck and the man slides one leg between hers, while placing his hands around her waist.

● Still caressing, the woman raises her right thigh and slides it toward her partner's waist. The man grips her thigh firmly and bends his knees to enable the woman to climb up him.

● The woman grips the man firmly behind the neck and he clasps his hands behind her back. With her right thigh wrapped around the man's back, the woman simply lifts her other leg to straddle her partner.

● At this point the man is ready and able to enter the woman as she wraps her legs around his back. He keeps his knees bent to support her weight, and she will need to hold on to his shoulders to help him balance.

climb ▶ lift ▶ balance ▶

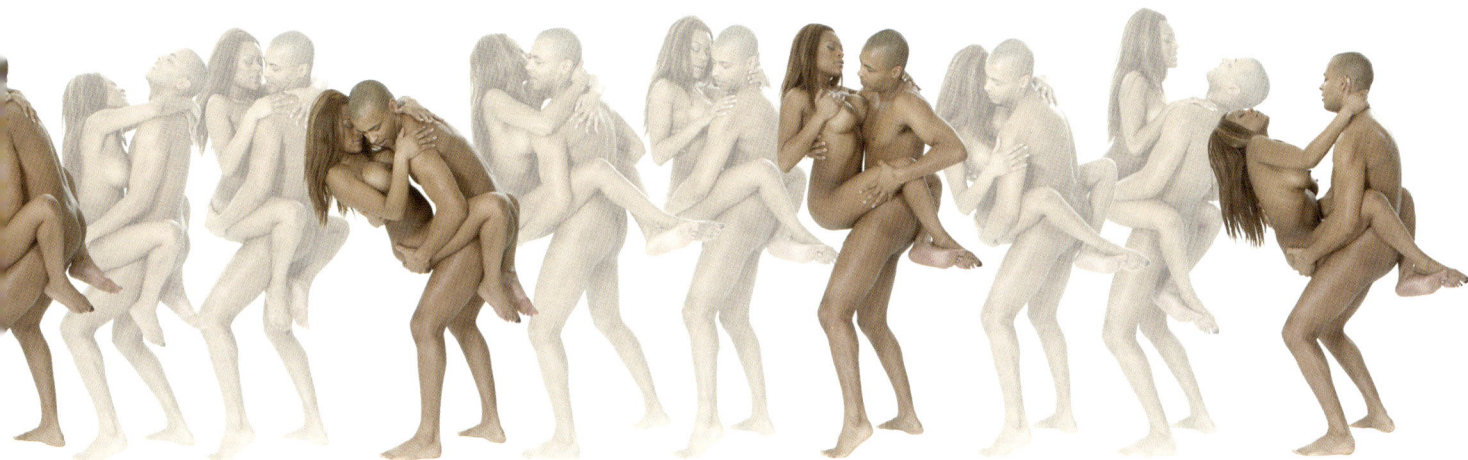

● In this position, the woman can hoist herself up and down, effectively stimulating her partner's penis inside her. She should be able to achieve good pressure on her clitoris too by rubbing against his pubic bone.

● To vary the tempo, the man leans forward, making sure that the woman is holding on to him tightly. He can also place his hands under her buttocks to help her get a good grip.

● Decide between you who is going to orgasm or you can both try for it. Although you will have good fun trying, you are unlikely to reach a satisfactory orgasm in this position because it requires so much strength.

● If the man tires, he can always lean the woman back against a wall. Both of you may be better able to orgasm in this position as it provides more pressure and friction.

grapevine II

This alternative version of the grapevine is slightly less exhausting for the man.

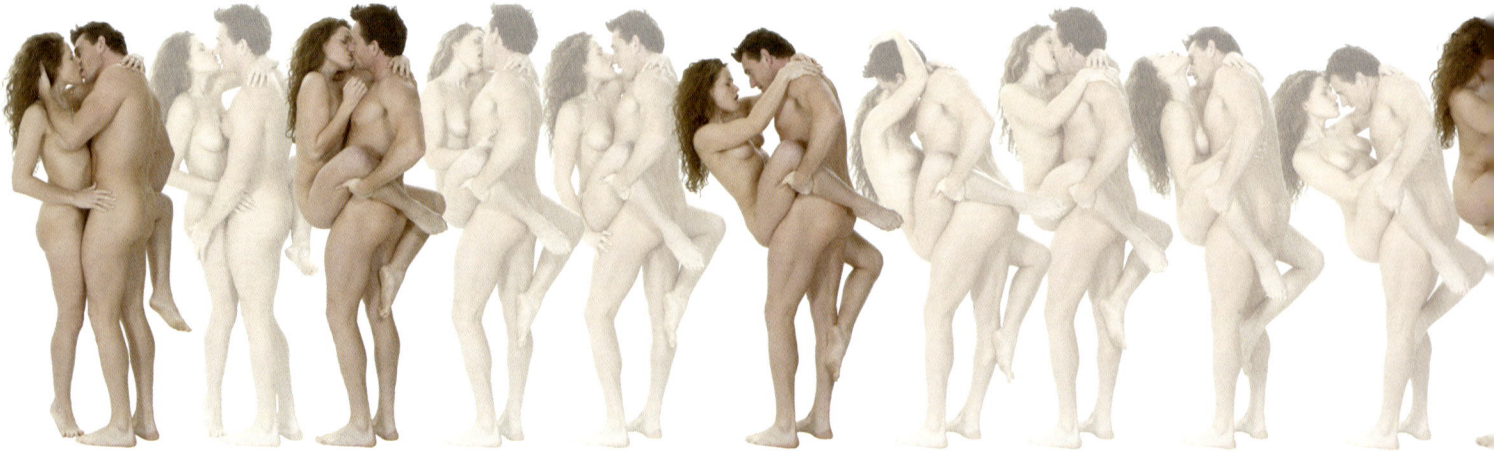

● The couple stand facing each other and embrace. They should both be excited from foreplay and ready for energetic lovemaking.

● As the woman raises her left leg and swings it around the man's waist, he grips her buttocks and lifts her right leg. He helps her wrap her right leg around his waist and takes hold of her thighs firmly.

● At this stage the man can enter the woman, while she grips him tightly around the back of his neck. Kiss each other deeply and enjoy the intimacy of this position.

● If the man keeps a firm hold on his partner's thighs, he can maneuver her up and down. She matches his rhythm by hauling herself up on his shoulders.

hold ▶ be intimate ▶ rhythm ▶

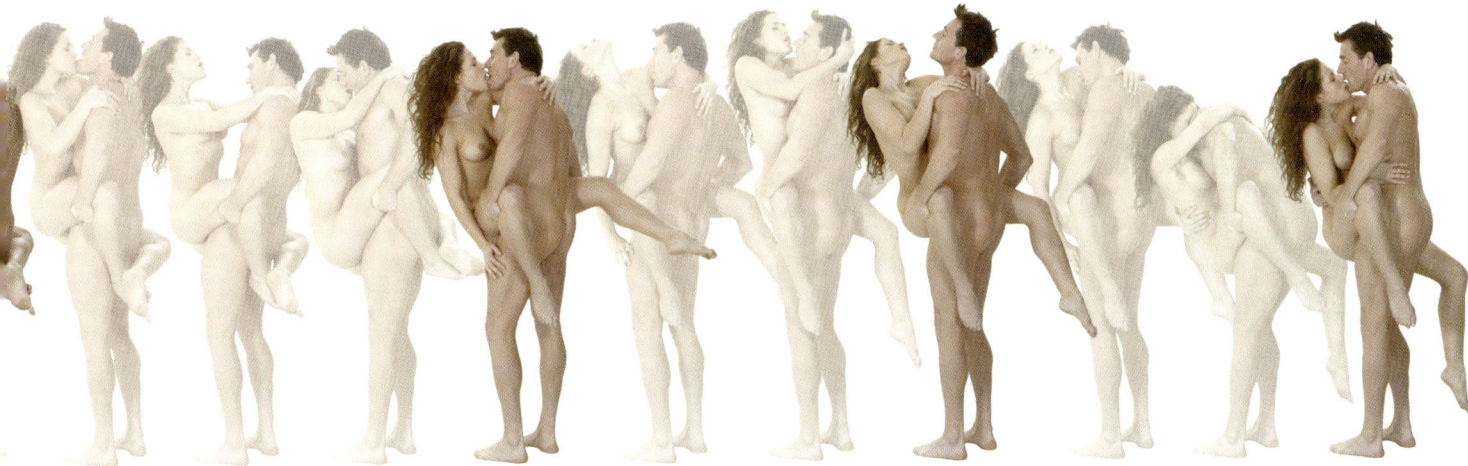

● The woman should be able to reach down and run her nails up and down the man's thigh to stimulate him. Remember to take time out to kiss, be intimate, caress each other, and be in love as much as making love.

● Although this position is quite tiring, once you have found a steady rhythm you can often reach orgasm, although not at the same time.

● If the man comes first, he will need a good reserve of strength and energy to remain standing and bear the woman's body weight while she reaches her orgasm.

● This will not be a problem if the woman comes first, but she too must be able to hang on so that her partner can orgasm. If you both get too tired, simply try another position in which to continue your lovemaking.

in the chair

standing positions

If you find standing positions very tiring, this position will be of interest since it gives you

all the benefits without the need for great strength.

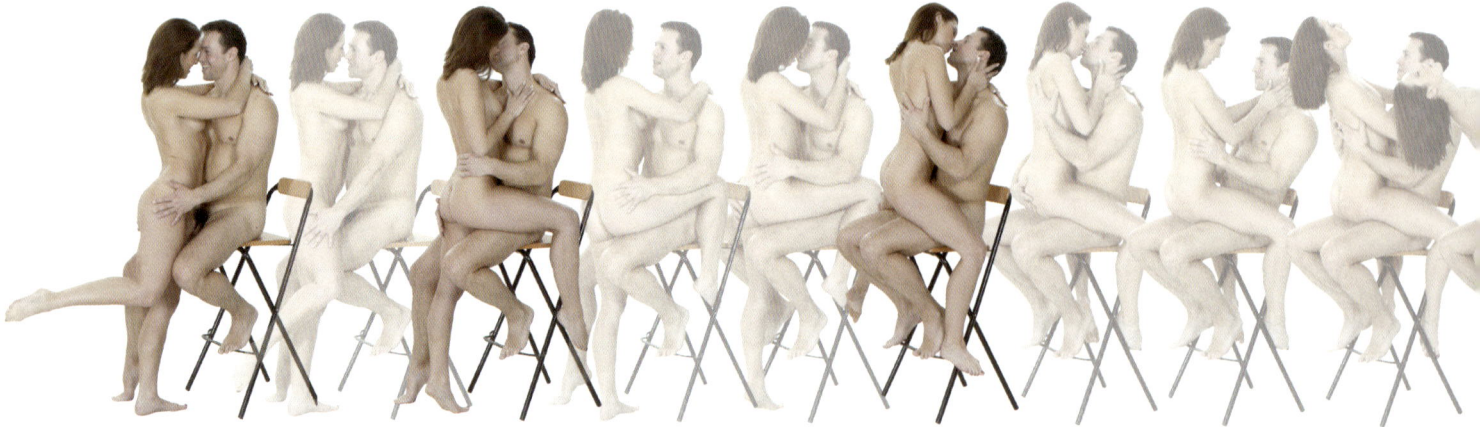

- You will need to find a chair that can take the strain. Choose something substantial that is not likely to collapse under your combined weight.

- The man sits on the chair and the woman sits astride his lap. Slowly she slides up toward him and they kiss deeply.

- The woman carefully maneuvers herself so that she is directly above the man's erect penis. She then pushes her body down hard so that her partner slides straight into her.

- If the woman rests her legs outside of the man's, then they should both find this position relaxing and not too tiring. This is a very intimate position and well designed for kissing.

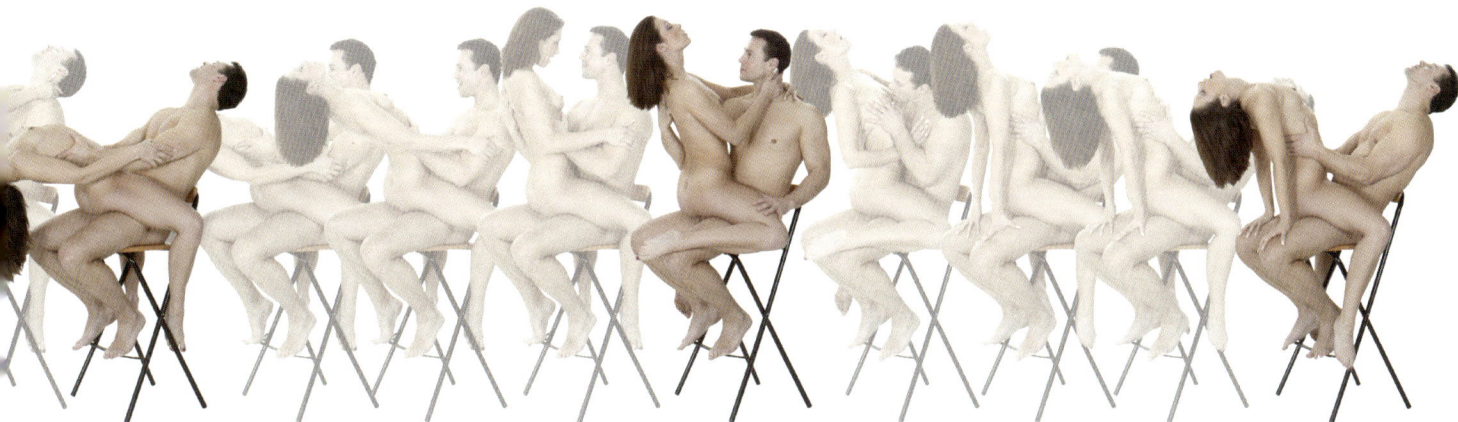

● In this position, the man can suck and lick his lover's breasts while he is making love with her. If she leans back to make her breasts stand proud, the man can squeeze them and suck her nipples comfortably.

● To reach orgasm in this position, the couple simply rock backward and forward. For leverage, the man lifts his feet until they are on tiptoe.

● If you find that this movement is not enough to achieve orgasm, stay in this position and stimulate each other with your hands for better results.

● If the chair has a bar across its legs, the man can rest his feet on it to give him extra purchase. This will help both of you to orgasm more easily.

on the kitchen table

Raunchy sex on the kitchen table usually finds a place on most people's list
of favorite fantasies. So why not go for it right now?

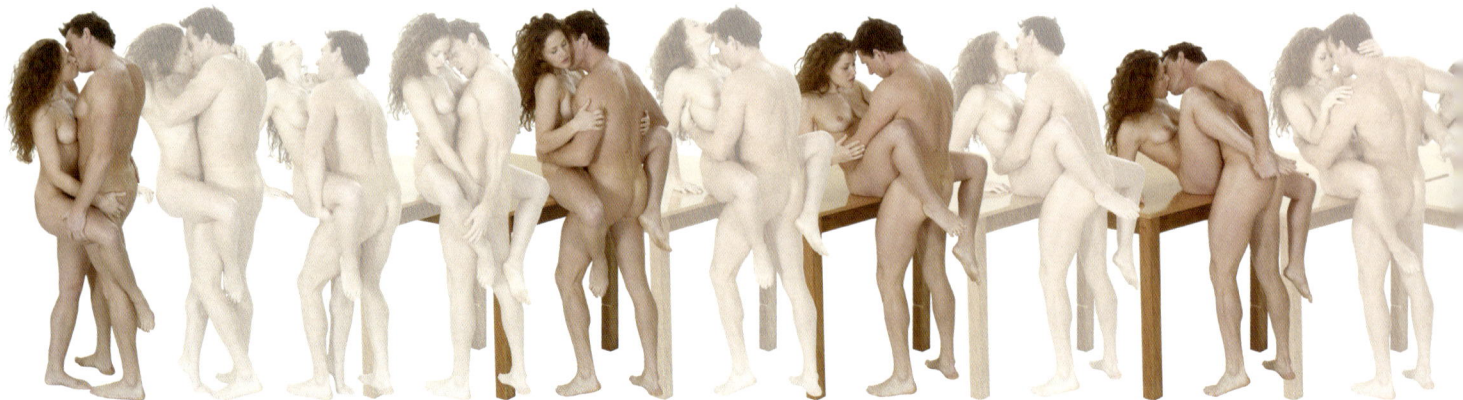

● Use a table that is strong enough to
take the weight of you both. Nothing
more could spoil the mood than the
table collapsing just as you reach
orgasm. Clear away any items that
might get knocked over or broken.

● The man leads the woman to the
table and helps her to get on it. At the
same time, he can glance over her
shoulder to check the area is clear
before they engage in heavy petting.

● If the table is at the right height, the
man enters the woman while she sits
on the edge. It is more likely that the
man will need to stand on a cushion
or some books to reach his partner.

● This is a really good position for
face-to-face intimacy, with kissing,
stroking, licking, and biting. It is also a
good position for quick raunchy sex,
perhaps a "quickie" after the kids have
gone to bed.

forethought ▶ **right height** ▶ **be spontaneous** ▶

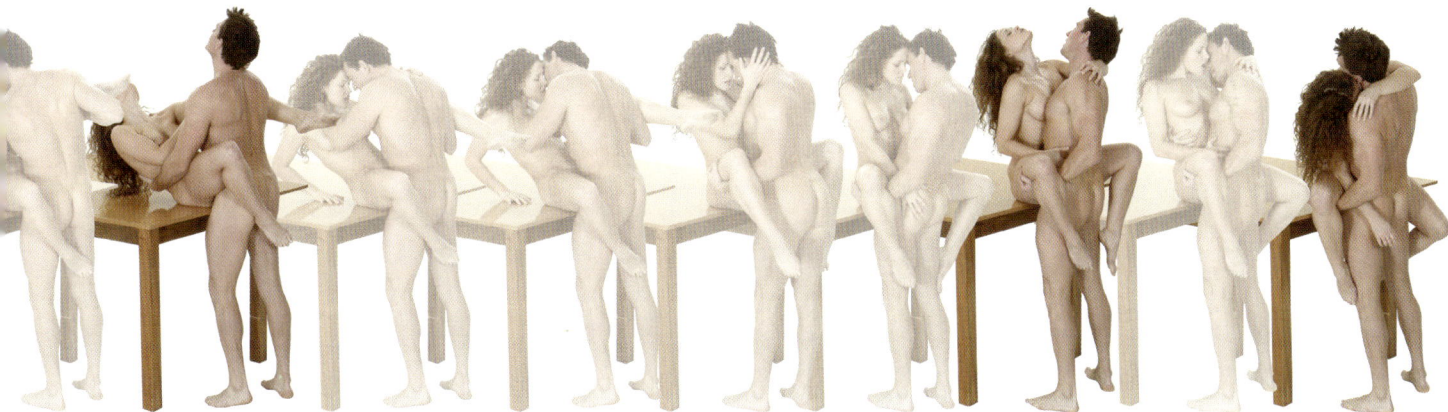

● The man has good access to the woman's clitoris, so if she needs further stimulation to reach orgasm he can stroke and rub her while he continues making love.

● Remember, if you are going to have wild and raunchy sex in the kitchen, it is best to make sure that the door is locked or at least that you cannot be disturbed. Imagine the kids or your mother walking in on you.

● Even during the raunchiest of sex, make some time for a little gentle lovemaking when you kiss and cuddle, be intimate and love each other.

● The great thing about having wild sex in the kitchen is that wine and food are close at hand after you have both had your orgasm.

the wheelbarrow

Of all the sexual positions that you can try, this one must be one of the most strenuous and athletic. But it is also one of the most fun and offers the deepest penetration.

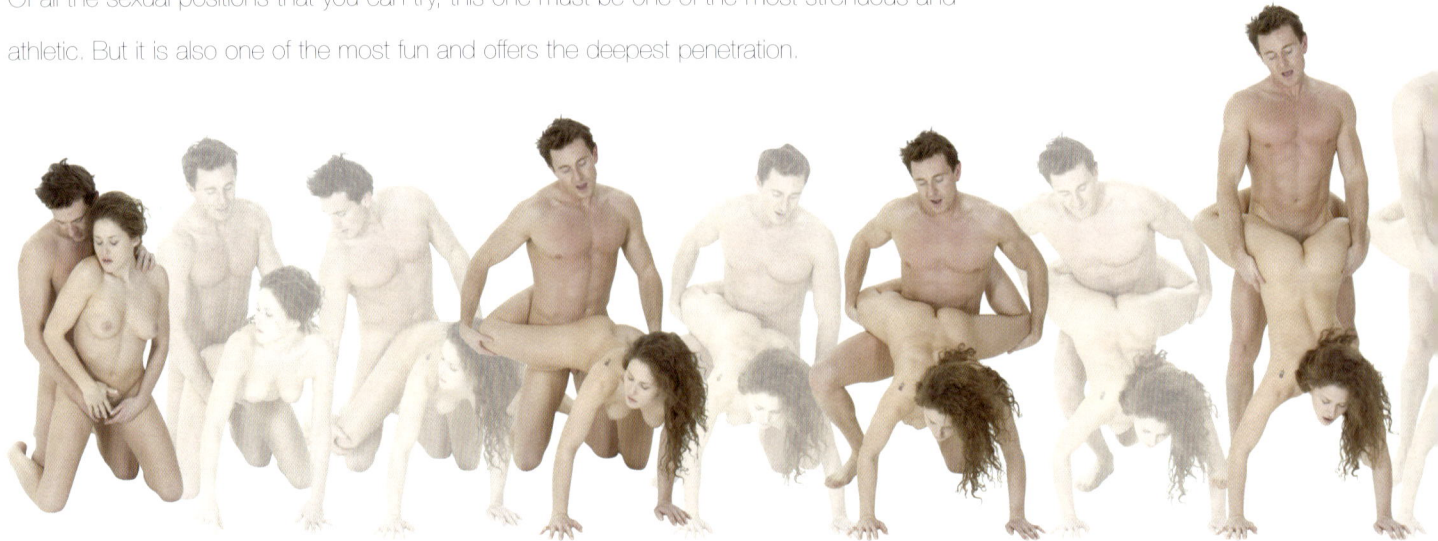

● The couple start in the kneeling position, with the man behind the woman and his legs inside hers. In this position they can fondle each other.

● Using her arms for support, the woman leans forward so that the man can enter her from behind. Some couples prefer to wait until the woman is in the full wheelbarrow position before the man enters her.

● The man takes hold of his partner's lower thighs, one at a time, and wraps them around his waist. The woman continues to support her weight on her hands, with palms facing down.

● Holding on tightly to her legs, the man slowly raises himself onto his feet. If he is strong enough this can be done in one swift go. If not, his attempts may result in a lot of falling over, much giggling, and plenty of fun.

■　　　　　　　　**lean forward**　▶　**strength**　▶　**have fun**　▶

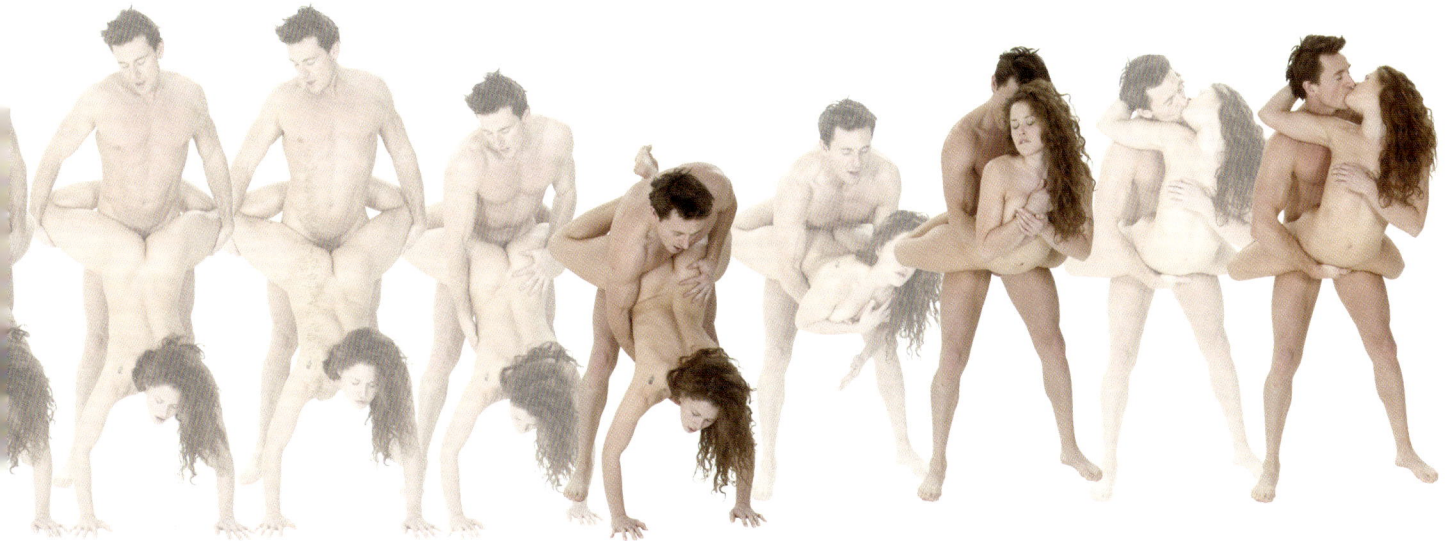

● Once he is standing up, the man can enter his partner, holding her upright with his hands on her thighs. Much of the woman's weight can be transferred to her legs wrapped around his body.

● The next stage of this position requires considerable strength and agility, so do not attempt it unless you are both very fit and healthy.

● The man leans forward and grips the woman around the belly with one hand. At the same time he levers her upright, placing a supporting hand on her buttocks, and she flips herself up into his arms.

● In this position they can kiss and the man can fondle his lover's breasts. Whether you can achieve orgasm depends entirely on your fitness levels!

be careful

bending and straightening

This is a great position for men who like to enter their partner from behind. It's not, however, all about his enoyment, as it allows the woman a great deal of pleasure too.

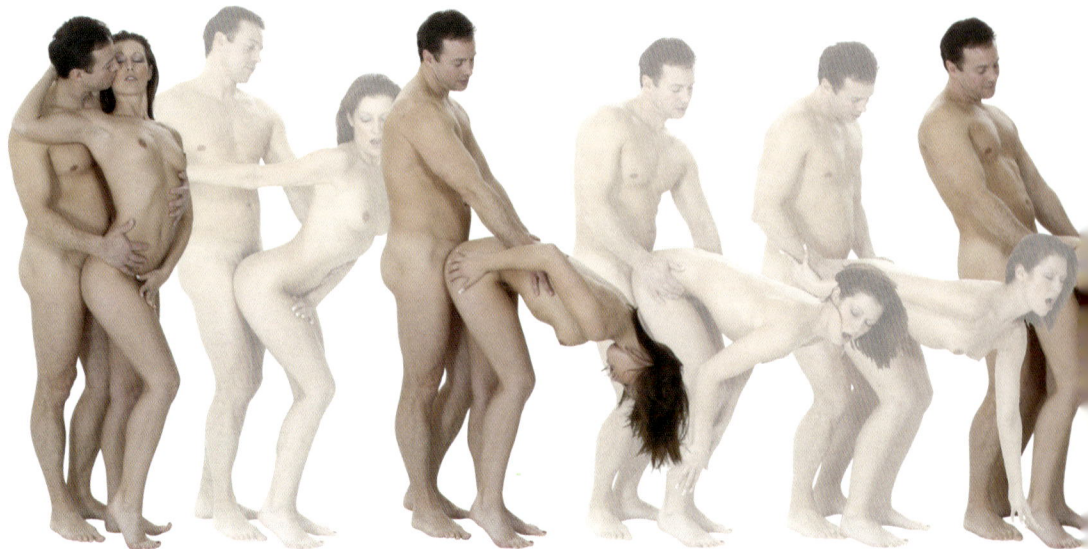

- The couple start in the standing position with the woman's back facing her lover. The man reaches forward to caress and excite her, while she presses her buttocks against his erection to increase his excitement.

- The woman then bends forward in an exaggerated way to stimulate her partner by pushing back hard against his groin.

- As the the man enters her from behind, the woman continues to bend toward the floor to enable him to penetrate her deeply.

- The woman places her hands on the floor for support and the man grips her around the waist so that they can thrust hard against each other. You can achieve orgasm either independently or simultaneously.

push back ▶ deep penetration ▶ thrust hard ▶

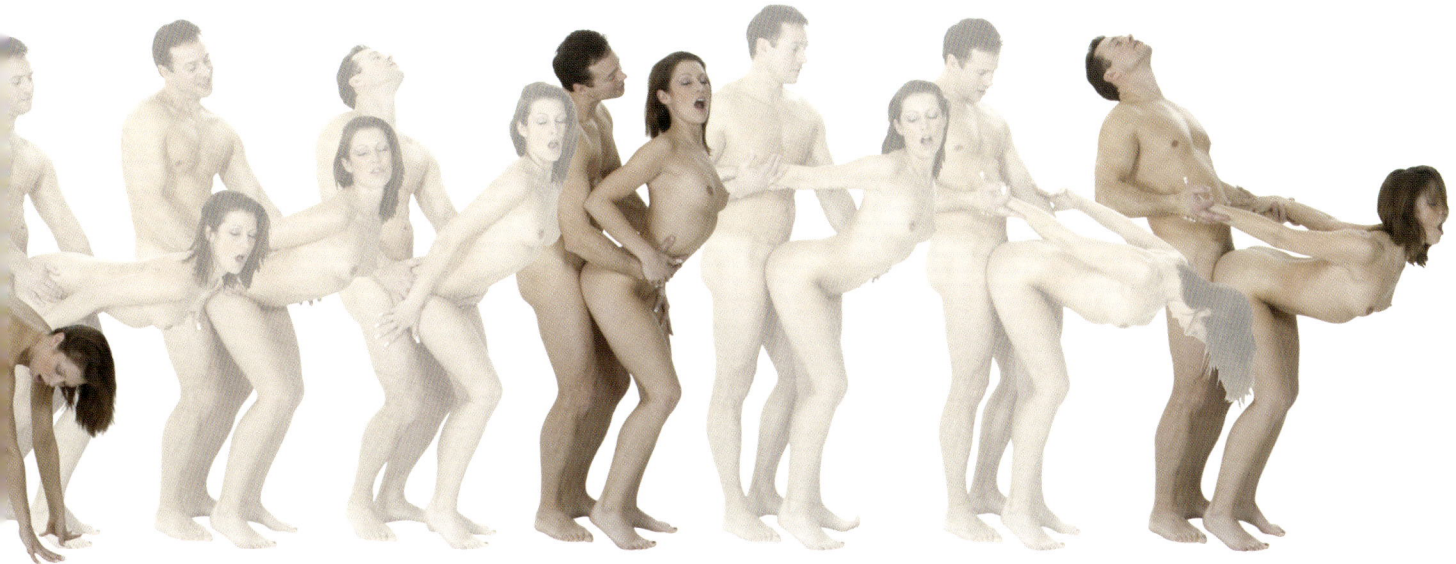

● If the couple do not reach orgasm, the woman can slowly straighten up. This places internal pressure on the man's erection which he will find stimulating and exciting.

● The woman can then alternate between bending and straightening her body, keeping in rhythm with his thrusts. By reaching behind to pull on his thighs, she can increase the force.

● At the next stage, the woman lifts her arms behind her and the man grips her hands in his. This allows you to pull and push against each other, with the woman arching her back.

● The man will probably be able to orgasm in this position. If the woman does not reach a climax, she will at least receive a lot of satisfaction.

straighten up ▶ **alternate** ▶ **pull and push** ▶ **II**

upside-down woman

This position can be hard on the woman's neck and spine, so it should only be attempted if she is fit, athletic, and healthy—as well as being a bit of a contortionist.

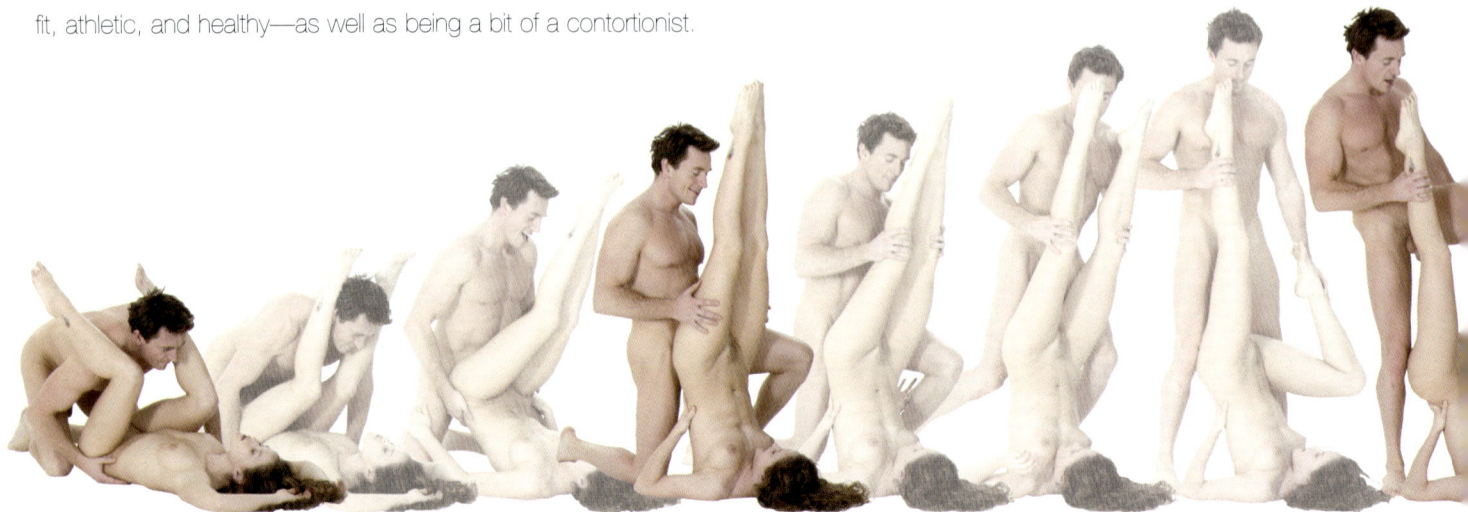

● The woman lies on her back and should relax into the position. The man then crouches between the woman's legs, letting her ankles rest behind his ears, and tucks his hands under her buttocks.

● The man slowly rises to his feet, supporting the woman's lower body as she pulls herself up into a shoulder-stand. The woman places her hands on her lower back for support and presses her shoulders into the floor.

● As the woman gets into the shoulder stand, the man slides his hands down her thighs and reaches to take hold of her shins. Once he is standing upright, he pulls her up so that she is in a full shoulder stand.

● Pushing one of the woman's legs to the side, the man steps over to stand in between her legs, making sure not to step on her head. The woman continues to support herself, keeping her hands on her lower back.

■   **stand up slowly** ▶   **shoulder stand** ▶   **step through** ▶

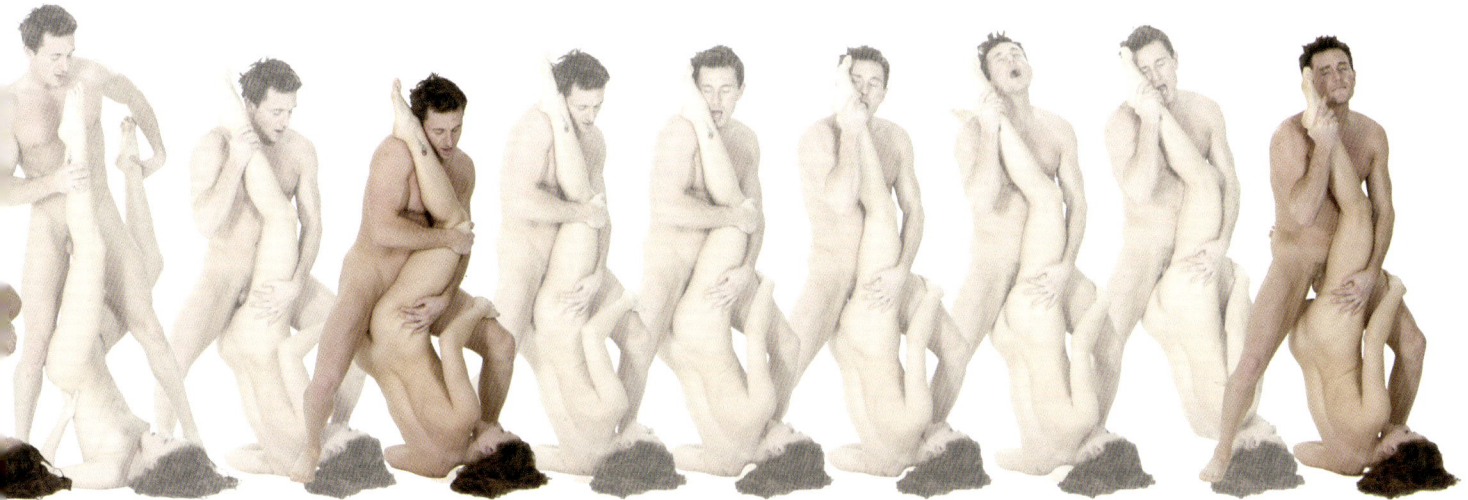

● Running his hands along her legs and thighs, the man slowly bends his knees and crouches down. The woman now starts to turn to one side.

● The woman reaches up to seize hold of the man's thigh to help take the pressure off her neck. At this point the man is ready to enter her and they can begin to make love.

● This position does not provide deep penetration, but it can be indulged in as a male fantasy when the mood takes you and provided that you feel athletic and energetic.

● Rather than for intercourse, this position is more for frotting (rubbing sexually against each other), and by this means orgasm may be achieved. Worth a try, if only once.

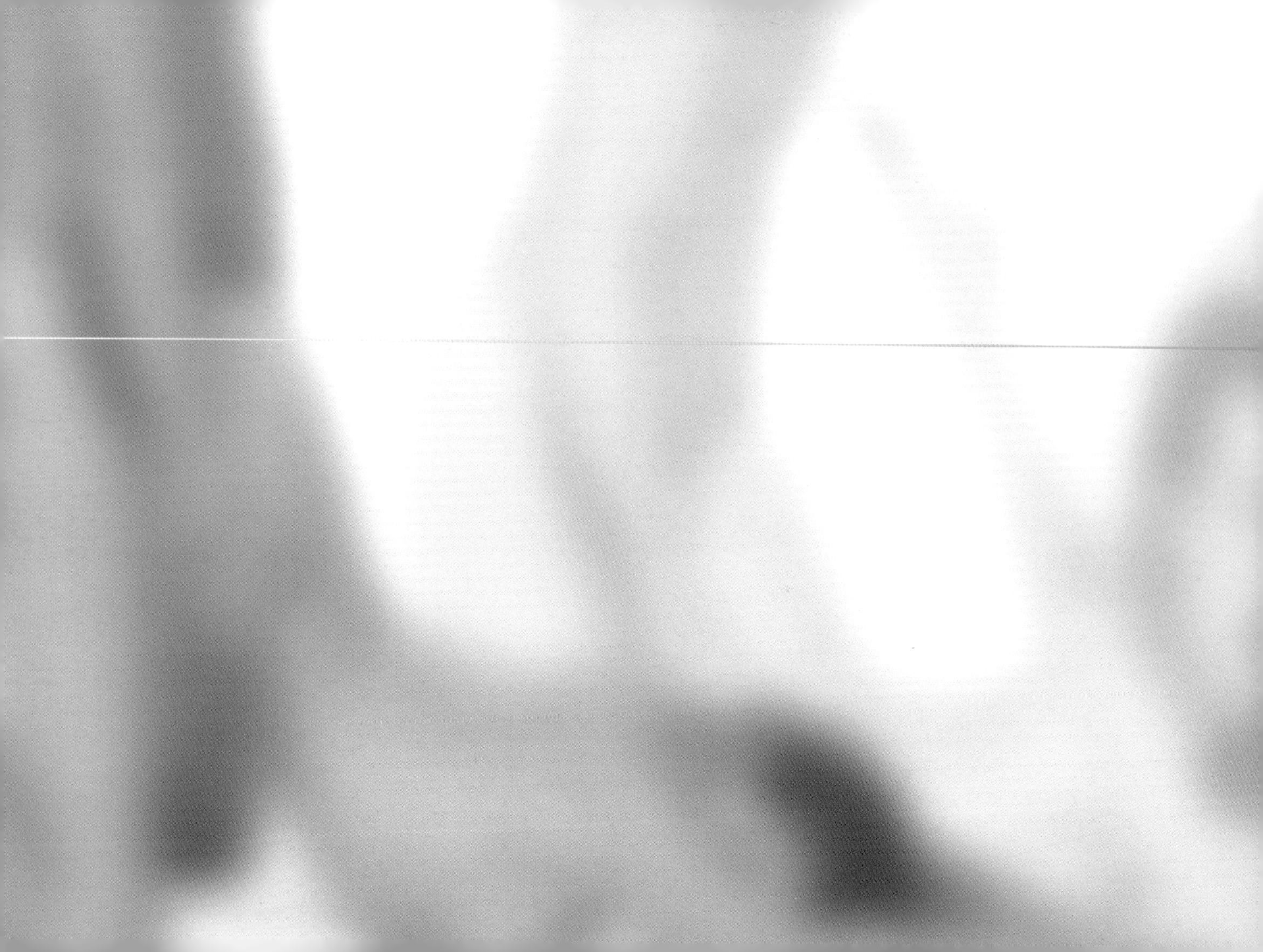

kneeling positions

from behind *kneeling positions*

Kneeling down with the man entering the woman from behind is a classic sex position and one that is a firm favorite with many couples.

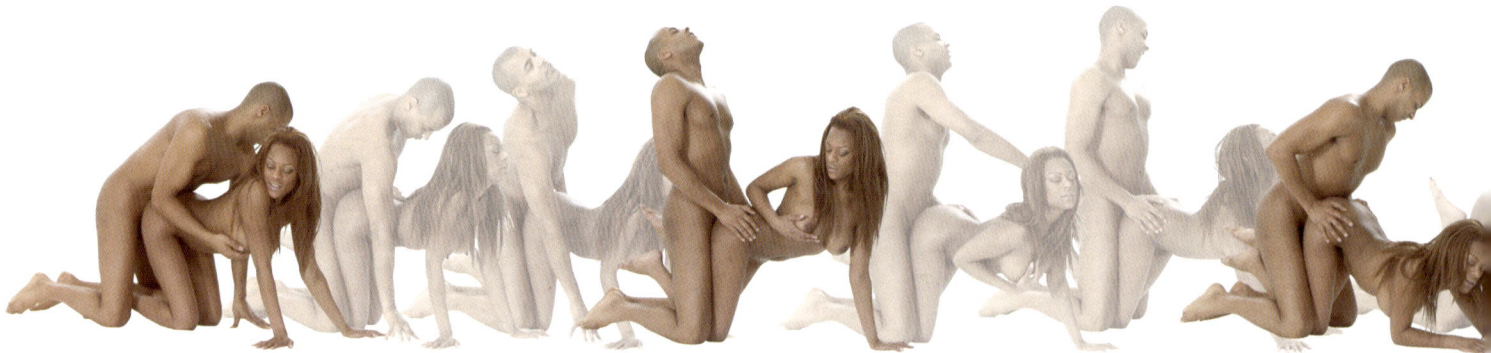

● The couple kneel together, with the woman's back facing the man. The pressure of her buttocks on his erection and his heavy thrusting on her buttocks, anus, and perineum is intensely stimulating for both of them.

● The couple have plenty of scope to play with each other in this position. The woman plays with her nipples to excite the man and to stimulate herself, and the man reaches forward to fondle the woman's breasts as well.

● This kneeling position is good for thrusting. The man can pull on his partner's hair, if she likes that, and the woman can alter the angle at which he enters her by raising or lowering her head from or to the floor.

● The man grips her buttocks and pushes and pulls them in time with his thrusts. As the woman alters the angle of her vagina, he can keep pace with her by leaning forward or backward.

■   **mutual stimulation** ▶   **thrust** ▶   **rhythm** ▶

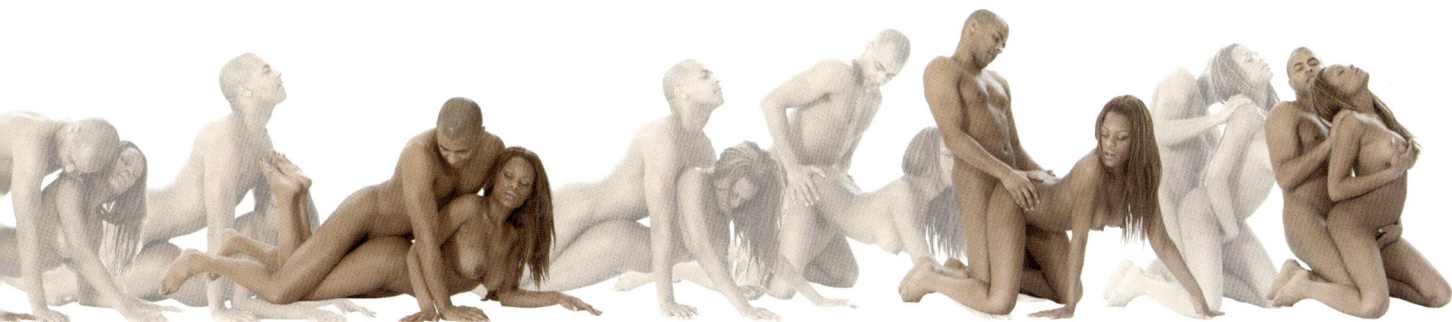

● The woman can slide down onto the floor while the man continues to make love to her. He will need to support his body weight on his arms so that he does not crush his partner.

● The woman twists from side to side to give the man access to her breasts and to enable her to push her buttocks harder against his groin.

● When she feels ready, the woman comes up onto her knees again and the couple continue making love in the kneeling position. By arching her back, the woman intensifies the force of her buttocks against his groin.

● If the woman pushes herself upright, she can masturbate her clitoris, allowing the couple to achieve orgasm together. This is one of the key reasons why this position is so popular.

take the weight ▶ **twist** ▶ **intensify** ▶ II

half kneeling, half lying

This is one of the many variations to be explored in the man-kneeling-behind-his-lover positions.

To begin with, it is less tiring than some of the other kneeling positions shown, and the position

is more comfortable for the woman, making it very suitable for pregnant women.

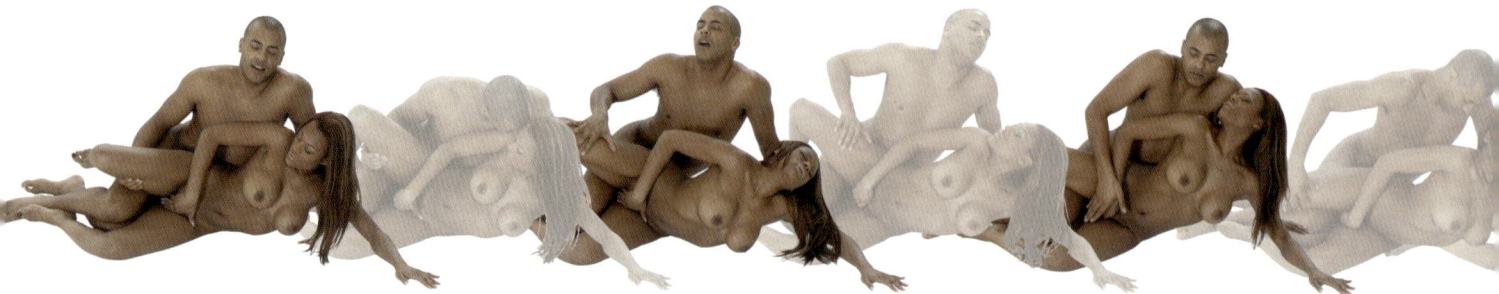

● The woman lies on her side and raises one leg in the air so the man can half-kneel, half-lie behind to enter her. The woman can easily reach her clitoris to masturbate in this position.

● Take the opportunity to kiss and be intimate and close. This position is easy on the woman and is very popular during the later stages of pregnancy.

● The man times his thrusts in rhythm with the woman stroking her clitoris. To stimulate his partner, the man strokes her thighs and she presses her buttocks back against his groin.

● The man reaches forward to caress her breasts. If the woman is in the throes of her orgasm, he can push hard against her hand as she masturbates herself.

■ be intimate ▶ rhythm ▶ orgasm ▶

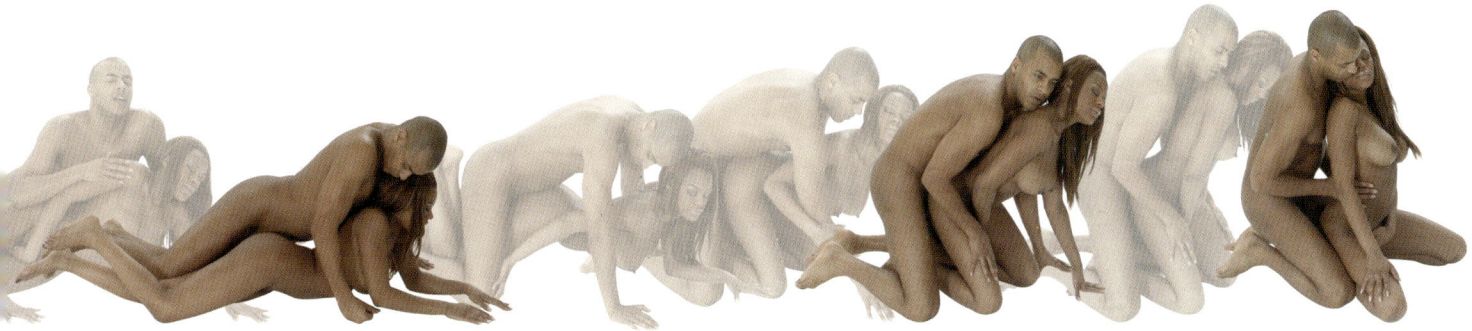

● Once her orgasm is over, it is the man's turn, and the woman can help him by rolling over onto her belly. Most men find this position very erotic and one in which it is easier to reach orgasm.

● If she is not heavily pregnant, the woman can rise onto her knees and push very hard back against his groin as he thrusts into her.

● As the man achieves orgasm, the woman reaches between her legs to rub his penis as it pushes into her. She then reaches down to caress his testicles and squeeze them as he ejaculates inside her.

● Once the man's orgasm subsides, the couple are in a good position to cuddle and be close. They can continue to be intimate and kiss each other lovingly.

his turn ▶ thrust ▶ rub ▶ ‖

more kneeling techniques

Several variations on the kneeling positions depend on whether the man's legs are outside or inside
the woman's legs and on how much the woman raises herself up on her knees.

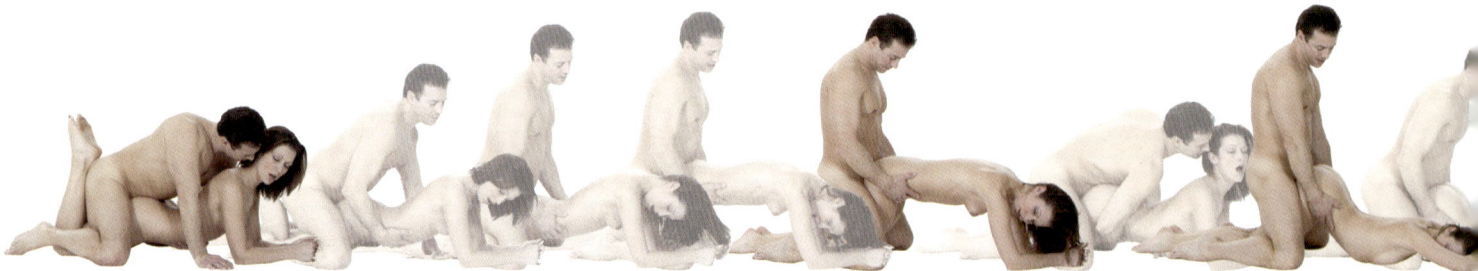

● Most men prefer to place their legs
outside the woman's, but the opposite
is true for many women. They get
more satisfaction when the man's legs
are placed in between theirs.

● The couple start in the easiest
position, with the woman lying face
down and the man kneeling astride
her back. As he enters his partner, the
man lovingly strokes and caresses her
back and neck.

● Once the man is inside her, the
woman thrusts hard against his groin
and raises herself onto her knees. If
she can orgasm in this position, she
can intensify the sensation by lowering
her head, causing a rush of blood.

● The man helps her to reach orgasm
by taking hold of her waist and pulling
her buttocks upward. This allows him
to stroke her clitoris and lets her
thrust backward to stimulate him.

stroke ▶   intensify ▶   masturbate her ▶

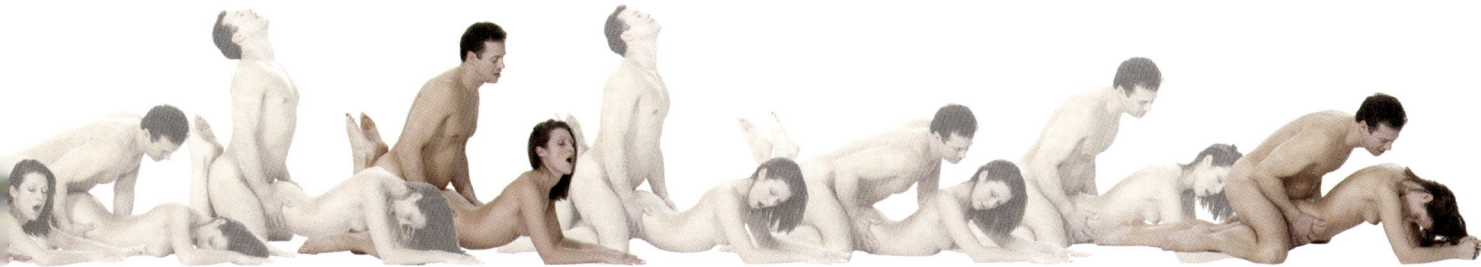

● The woman may need to collapse after her orgasm, but the man can remain inside her, moving very gently with tiny thrusts to keep his own passion going. This will not disturb her diminishing orgasmic feelings.

● When the woman is ready, the man can slowly increase the tempo of his thrusts to reach orgasm. The woman lowers her buttocks to increase the pressure against his groin by pressing her forearms into the floor.

● As he ejaculates inside her, the man keeps stroking and caressing his partner while she continues thrusting against his groin. In this way, he is likely to retain his erection and the couple can continue lovemaking.

● Once they have both recovered and the man has kept his erection, the woman can raise herself onto her knees for more lovemaking. Alternatively, the couple can simply relax into being close and loving.

move gently ▶ **orgasm** ▶ **continue** ▶ II

face-to-face kneeling

Some kneeling positions require more agility than others. The position shown here is quite energetic, so you will have to be pretty fit—but it does allow for deep penetration to be achieved.

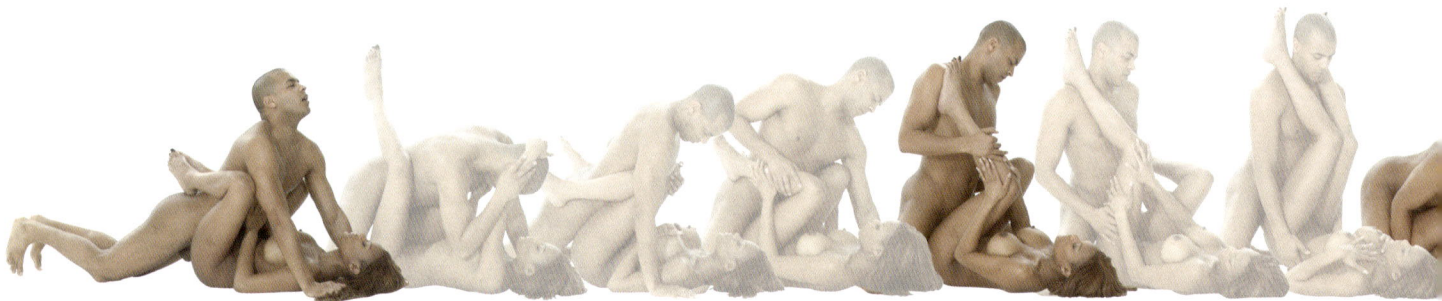

● If the couple are making love in the standard missionary position, it is quite easy to move into a kneeling position without the man having to withdraw from the woman.

● The man slowly lifts himself off his partner, drawing his knees up one by one and using his arms to support himself. The woman raises her legs so that he fits snugly against her groin.

● Kneeling, the man needs to press quite hard against the woman to hold his position, as it is easy for him to slip out doing this. The woman has good access to her clitoris and masturbates as the man thrusts into her.

● By raising the woman's legs up high so that her heels rest on his shoulders, the man will be able to enter his partner much more deeply.

■   snug fit   ▶   press hard   ▶   deep penetration   ▶

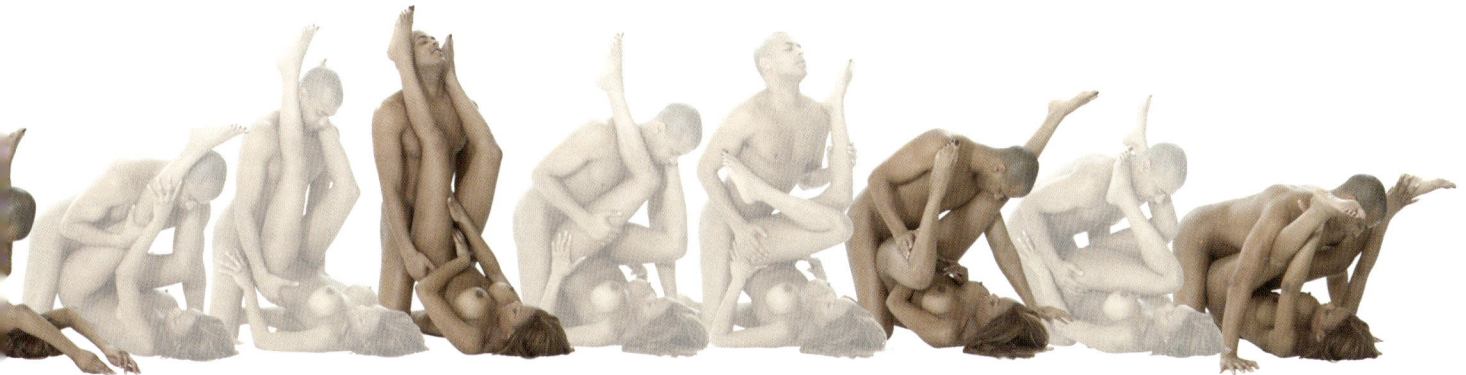

● With the man tilting forward so he is pressing down on her legs, the woman scissors his head between her knees, enabling him to achieve very deep penetration.

● If the woman now raises her legs as the man kneels upright, she can masturbate freely and he can orgasm if he is ready.

● If the couple are exploring anal sex, a fairly athletic woman can open her legs and raise her back so that only her shoulders are on the floor. This provides a very good position.

● Deeper penetration can be achieved if the woman opens her legs wide. This is highly recommended for men with a small penis, as it gives them the ability to satisfy their partner more effectively.

woman on top

from oral to on top

If the woman is giving the man pleasure with her mouth and he is lying down, it can be good to progress to full sex without him having to move too much. This transition is an easy solution if the woman wants him to come inside her.

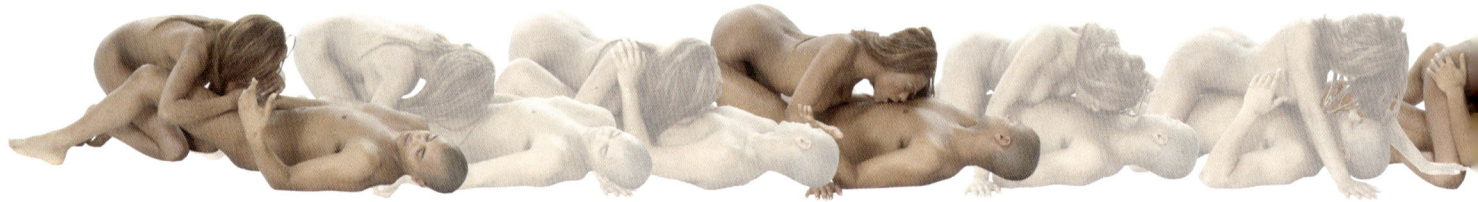

● The man lies down on his back and the woman performs oral sex on him by squatting between his legs and taking him in her mouth.

● When she senses that the man is close to orgasm, the woman continues sucking but leans forward at the same time so that she is ready to work her way up his body.

● The woman licks her way up her partner's body, licking and kissing his nipples on the way. She holds onto his penis and masturbates her partner so that his orgasm does not subside and he retains his erection.

● As the woman reaches a point where she can straddle the man, she helps him to enter her and lets him caress her breasts as she does so.

● To make the man reach orgasm, the woman leans backward and uses her thighs to move up and down on his penis. She continues caressing his chest at the same time.

● To further the man's excitement, the woman plays with her own breasts. This type of visual show is enjoyed by most men. She can also reach behind her and caress her partner's testicles.

● Placing her hands flat on the man's stomach or chest, the woman pushes herself to and fro with more pressure and force. In this way, the man can reach her clitoris and stroke it to help her come as well.

● Even if the man does not want to come, the couple can enjoy the woman being on top and share the pleasure of their intimacy.

caress   ▶   visual excitement   ▶   orgasm   ▶   II

woman on top

Most women find that they reach orgasm much more easily if they are on top of the man. This position gives them a greater measure of control and easier access to their clitoris for masturbation.

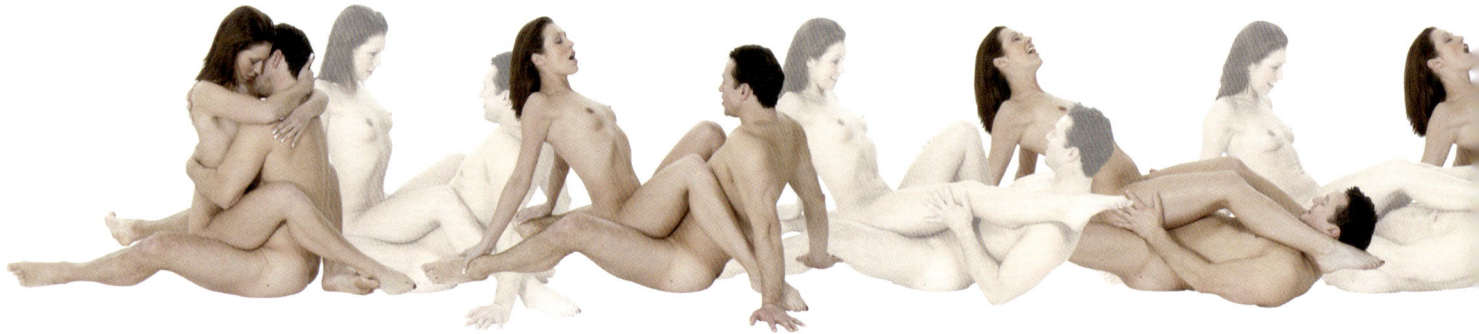

● The man sits on the floor and opens wide his outstretched legs. The woman, entwined around his back, sits astride his lap with her legs over his thighs. The man can achieve quite deep penetration as he enters her.

● The woman leans back, placing her hands behind her, with palms facing down to support her body weight. If the man now lifts his thighs off the floor, the couple can get good friction.

● If the woman raises her legs high enough, she can scissor his head with her ankles. The man presses his thighs tightly against her buttocks, allowing the couple to rock backward and forward to achieve orgasm.

● This is a very erotic experience for the man visually because he is able to watch his penis sliding in and out of his lover's vagina.

■　　　　　　　　friction　　　　▶　　　rock to and fro　　　▶　　　visual excitement　　　▶

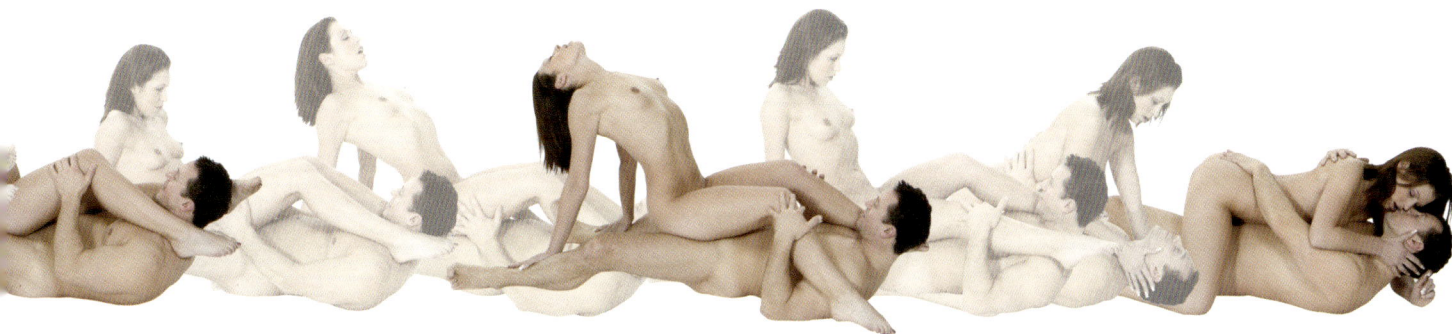

● By raising and lowering her hips, the woman exerts considerable pressure on her partner's penis. Squeezing him with her vaginal muscles, she should be able to bring him to orgasm with the minimum of effort.

● By leaning back to grip the man's ankles, the woman can confine his movements. Some men find this very mild form of bondage exciting.

● Try "soul drinking," an exciting practice recommended by Chinese Taoist sex treaties. Simply keep good eye contact as you each come and look deeply into your lover's eyes.

● As their orgasm subsides, the couple collapse onto each other. The woman gradually works her way up to the man's face where they can kiss intimately and be close to each other.

squeeze ▶ ▶ **eye contact** ▶ ▌▌

woman in charge

For some women, being totally in charge during sex is incredibly exciting. Plenty of men enjoy this too, since it takes away any need for them to worry about their performance.

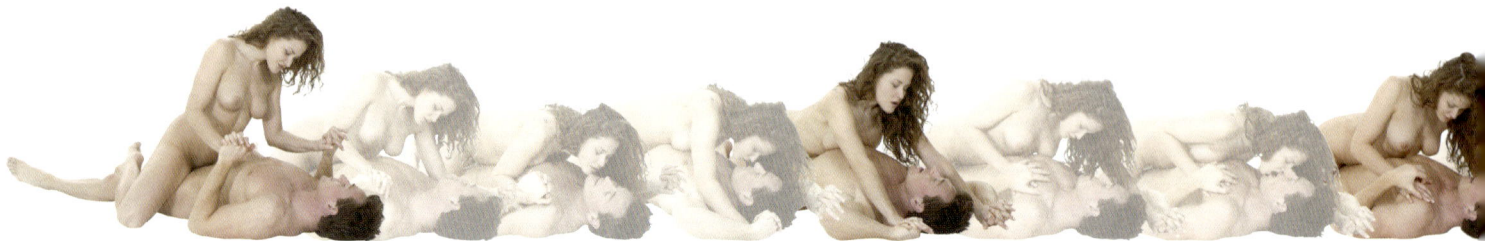

● If the man lies down, the woman can straddle him and hold his hands to restrict his movements. By locking her knees into the ground, she will restrict him even more.

● The woman leans forward and teases her partner by rubbing her breasts across his chest and face. She can also reach up to kiss him, still teasing and tempting him.

● As the man arcs his back, the woman rubs her groin across his erect penis. She does not let him enter her yet, so as to bring the teasing to an unbearable pitch.

● Still pinning him down, the woman kisses her partner deeply, letting her tongue gently excite him. He raises his head and begs her to let him enter her. The decision belongs to the woman because she is in charge.

tease ▶ tantalize ▶ dominate ▶

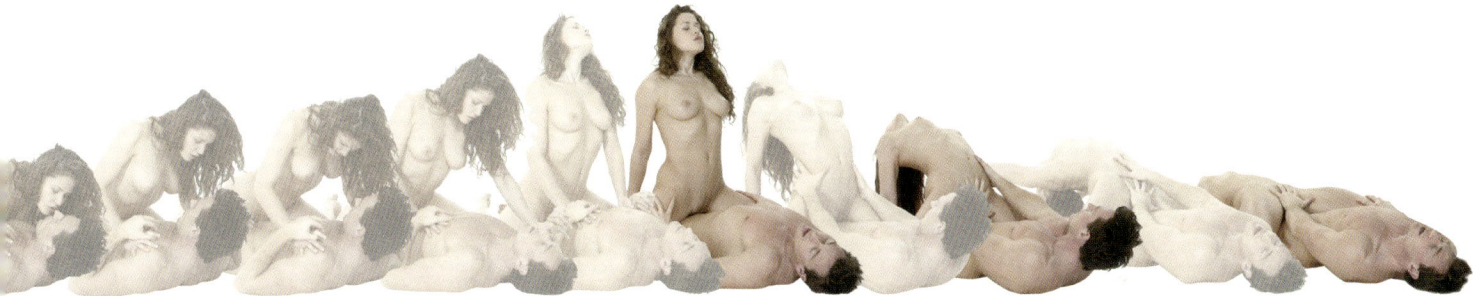

● Finally the teasing is over and the woman lets the man enter her. He pushes hard into her but she is still in control and dictates the pace. She can force the man back down by pushing firmly on his chest.

● When the woman is ready, she lets the man enter her fully. This is her turn, her orgasm, and he is the tool to be used to satisfy her. She straddles and rides him, setting her own rhythm.

● By leaning backward she exposes her clitoris to the man and allows him to stroke, rub, and fondle her, making her reach orgasm. She enjoys the sensation of him being deep inside her.

● As she orgasms the tension is too much for the man and he climaxes, ejaculating just as the woman comes. The couple collapse together on the floor, exhausted and satisfied.

the spinning top

This is a good position for the woman to be on top without the dominance seen in the previous position. Traditionally, it has always been known as the spinning top and it is easy to see why.

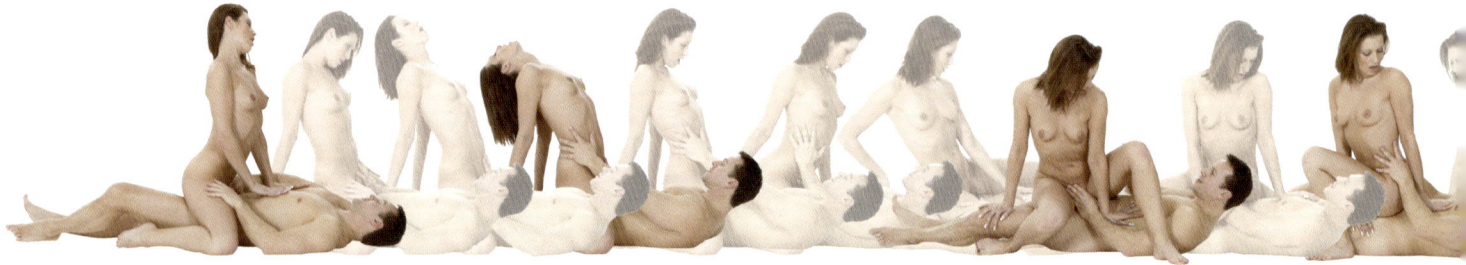

● The man lies on his back and the woman sits astride him across his waist. Her legs should be outside his, with her knees resting on the ground, so that he can enter her easily.

● The man has good access to her clitoris and can stimulate the woman if she leans backward, supporting her weight on her hands. In this position the couple can have great sex, but they can experiment further.

● It is important for the woman to take things slowly if she is to complete the spinning top without the man's penis falling out of her. She starts by raising her left leg off the floor.

● As she swings her left leg over the man's body, her right leg slides down over his feet. Turning slowly, she finds herself sitting at right angles to her partner and he is still inside her.

move slowly ▶ turn ▶

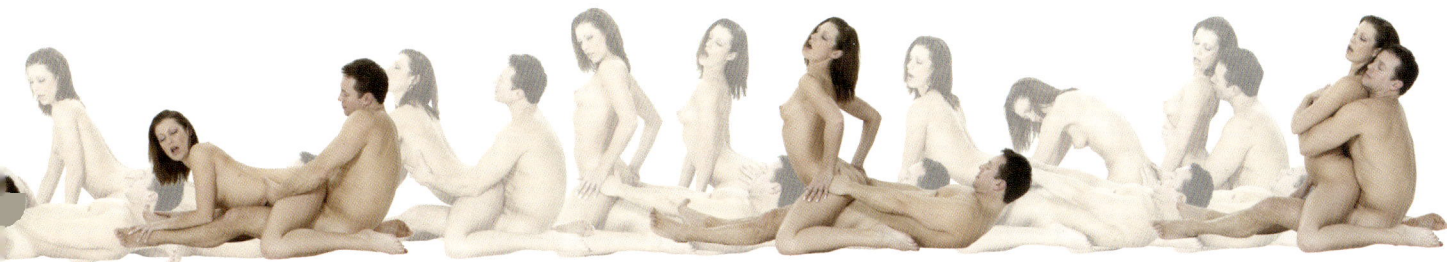

● With her next 90-degree turn, taking her right leg over the man's legs while her left leg slides down his, the woman gives the man a full view of her posterior. She flips her thighs back until they are alongside his buttocks.

● The woman is now astride her partner and sits upright. The man runs his hands up and down her buttocks while she masturbates her clitoris. Penetration in this position is very deep and satisfying for the couple.

● To help the man reach his climax, the woman alternates arching and relaxing her back to bring friction on his penis. With skill and experience, the woman can bring both of them to orgasm simultaneously.

● Once the couple have come, they can enjoy this position simply to relax together and to be close. They stay as they are, just holding each other.

visual excitement ▶ **deep and satisfying** ▶ **orgasm** ▶ **11**

lap dancing

This is a wonderful position if the couple feel energetic, sexy, and full of fun. It allows the woman complete freedom to be creative and orgasmic.

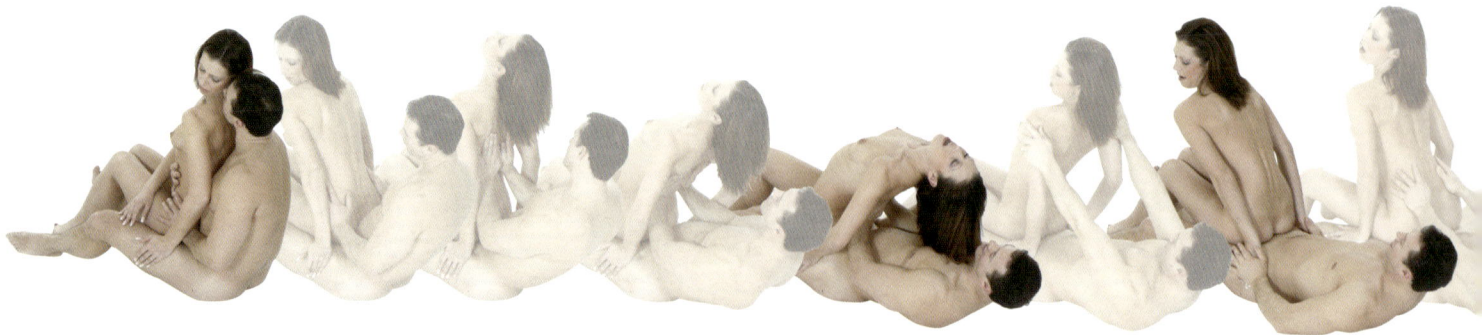

● The man sits down with his knees slightly raised and the woman sits in his lap with her legs inside his. This position allows deep penetration, and many women find it very satisfying.

● The man slowly lies back onto the floor, while the woman arches her back and grinds her buttocks hard against the man's penis. This makes her partner very excited.

● With the man now lying flat on the floor, the woman arches her back and lowers her head until it is touching his. The man reaches forward to caress the woman's breasts.

● He also holds on to her shoulders for extra purchase and thrusts hard into her. By placing her hands behind her, the woman can push down hard on the man's hips so that she can move up and down in rhythm.

grind ▶ caress ▶ rhythm ▶

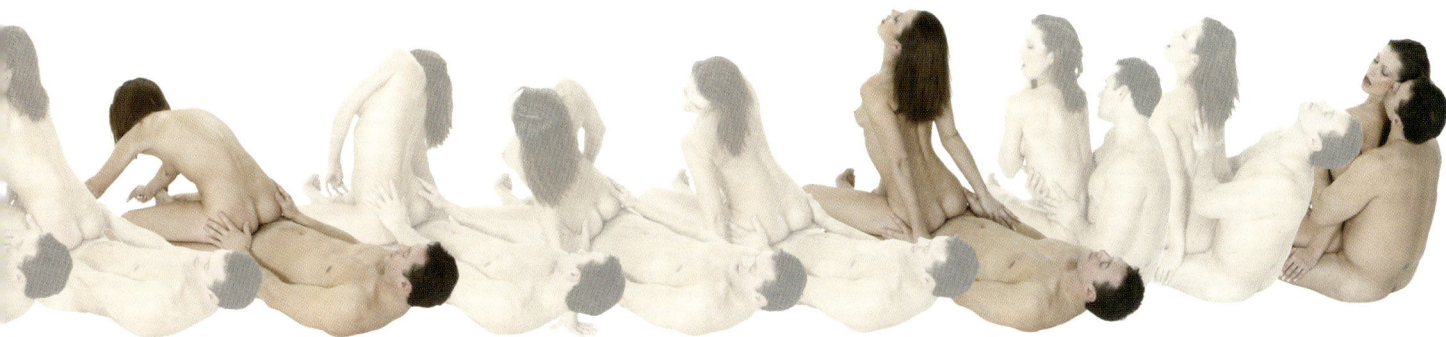

● As the woman starts to rock backward and forward in time with the man's thrusts, it feels like a dance. She can also rock from side to side or swivel in a circular movement, creating pressure on the man's penis inside her.

● As the woman swings to each side, sweeping close to the floor, the man lifts his buttock on the opposite side to increase the motion. The woman can use her hands for support to stop her and her partner from falling over.

● The couple hold hands and pull hard against each other to increase the tempo and tension. In this position the woman can grind her pubic bone against the man's penis.

● Both of the lovers, perhaps independently, are able to produce enough friction to reach orgasm in this position. If not, they will still get a lot of fun from trying it and will certainly burn up some energy.

woman pleasuring herself

In this position the pleasure belongs to the woman and she can make herself come easily and frequently. The man's role is to thrust as and when she needs the stimulation.

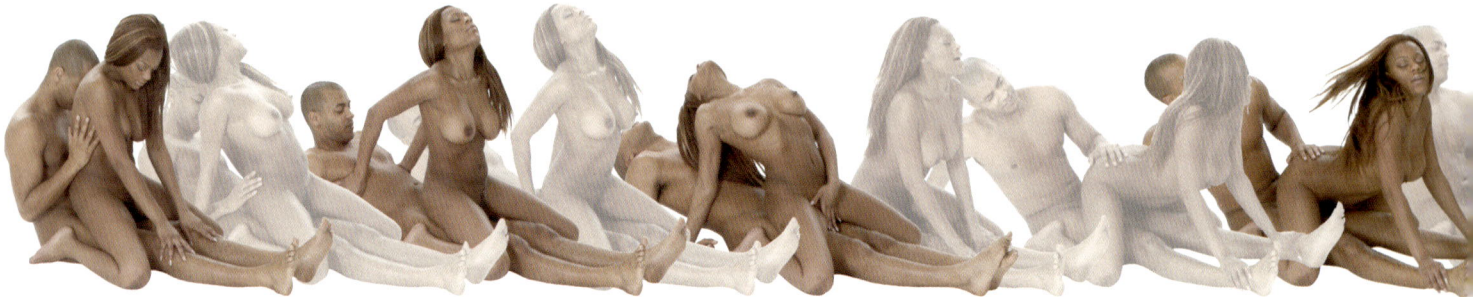

● The man sits on the floor with his legs outstretched in front of him. The woman kneels in his lap and leans backward so that the man can enter her and fondle her breasts.

● Staying in the kneeling position, the woman flexes her lower legs to raise herself up and down on his erect penis. This allows her to control the depth to which he enters her.

● The woman can reach her clitoris in this position. As the man thrusts into her, she strokes and rubs her clitoris, pleasuring herself to orgasm.

● By leaning forward to grip the man's ankles, the woman achieves greater control. The man takes hold of her buttocks to strengthen his thrusts.

control ▶ orgasm ▶ grip ▶

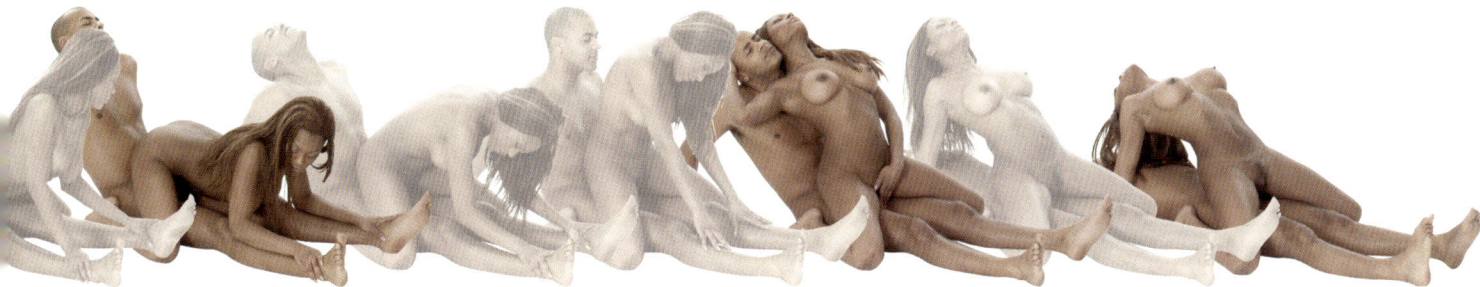

● The woman alternates arching and relaxing her back, rocking to and fro to increase her pleasure and control the depth of his penetration. She may find that shallow entry stimulates her more around her clitoris.

● If the woman keeps her lower legs well back and leans forward so that she is lying along the man's legs, she can caress his legs with her breasts, brushing them seductively against his skin. This also stimulates her nipples.

● By now the woman is close to orgasm and returns to stroking her clitoris to make herself come. The man braces himself against her and thrusts in time with her strokes.

● As his partner arches her back in orgasm, the man follows her lead, thrusting as suits her needs. He pushes up hard with his hips to give deeper and greater penetration as she comes.

stimulate ▶ **brush seductively** ▶ **coordinate** ▶ II

woman pleasuring the man

With practice and skill, the woman can make her partner come by sitting on his penis and pumping herself up and down. This is quite tiring for her but extremely exciting for him.

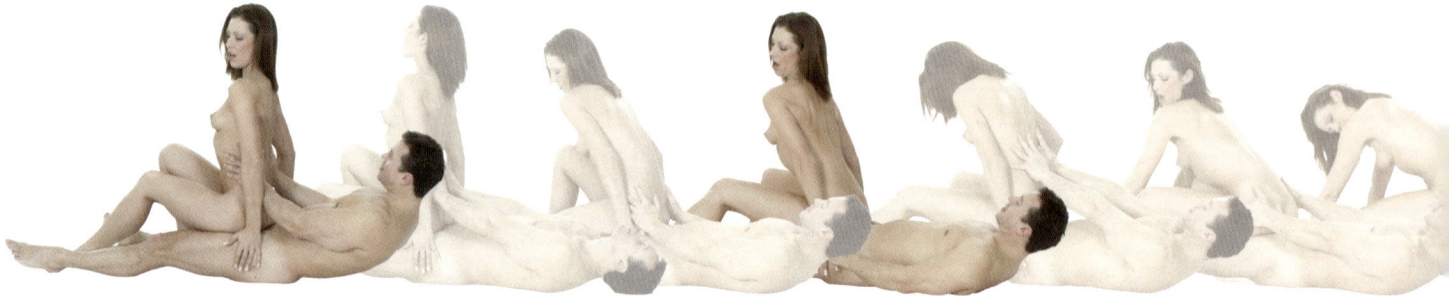

● The man lies back on the floor, guiding the woman onto his lap. Once she is sitting comfortably, he slowly enters her. She grips the sides of his hips to help her bounce up and down.

● The man grips his partner's buttocks as she bounces so that he can time his thrusts with her movements. The woman varies the depth of the man's penetration by sliding her legs forward.

● As the man thrusts into her, the woman lean forward to caress his testicles. He pushes hard against her back as she pleasures him.

● Leaning forward to grip the man's ankles, the woman presents her bottom to him for touching and feeling. This helps to increase his excitement.

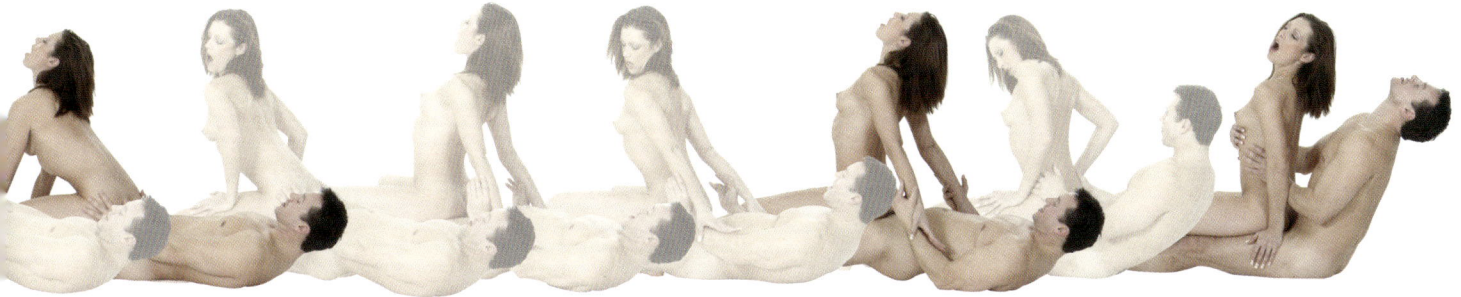

● Using her thigh muscles, the woman pumps up and down on her partner's penis. She places her hands on her thighs to strengthen her movements.

● If the woman reaches behind her and takes hold of the man's hands, the couple can thrust together in time. The woman rocks backward and forward to stimulate him further.

● This position is enjoyed by women who are capable of a vaginal orgasm, that is, without stimulating their clitoris. Although this exercise is designed for the man's pleasure, if the woman comes it will excite him even more.

● As the man comes, he reaches around the woman to caress her breasts. She forces herself hard down into him by gripping his thighs.

increase motion ▶ **thrust together** ▶ **his pleasure** ▶ **II**

face to face *on top*

In the face-to-face position, the woman is most definitely on top. She is in charge, in control, and very dominant. This position is fun, sexy, and very exciting for both partners.

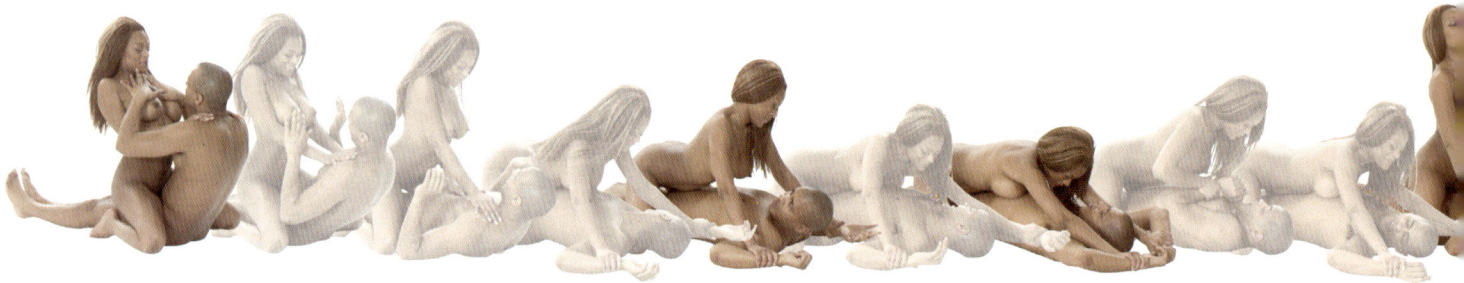

● The man sits down with his legs outstretched in front of him. The woman sits in his lap, facing him, with his penis inside her. The woman sets the pace, the tempo, and the rhythm.

● Leaning forward, the woman pins down her partner and teasingly holds his hands to stop him caressing her breasts. She grinds her pubic bone against him to further his excitement.

● This position is fun. You and your partner can laugh and enjoy the role-playing, being silly, and play-wrestling.

● Because the woman is half kneeling she can use her lower legs to control the depth and hardness of the man's thrusts. She is dominant and can tease him as much as she wants.

tease   ▶   **play**   ▶   **dominate**   ▶

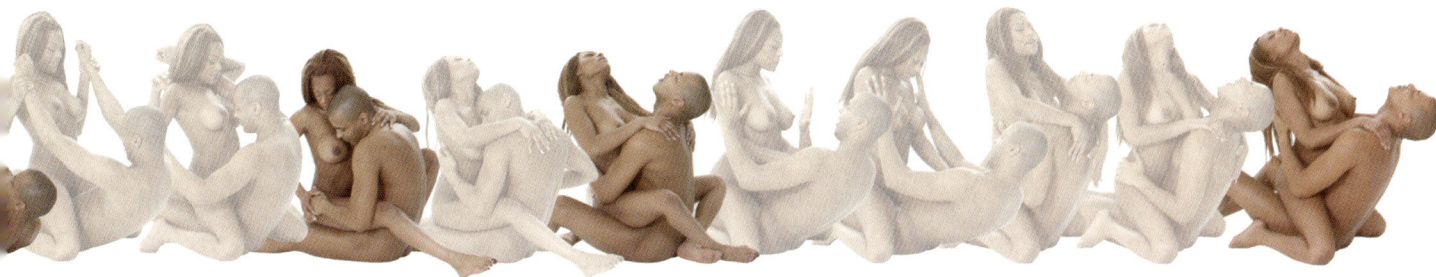

● The man tries to sit up and wrestle with his lover. He attempts to pin her down, but she is in charge and keeps her controlling position easily.

● The man caresses his partner's breasts, which will seem fuller and rounder because she is sitting upright. He buries his head between the breasts and sucks hard on her nipples.

● As she sits astride him, the woman pumps up and down on his penis to make him come. This requires a degree of fitness as it can be tiring on the leg muscles in particular.

● When the man comes, he should sit up so the woman can hold him tightly. She arches her back so that he can caress her breasts easily as he comes inside her.

control ▶ straddle ▶ ‖

scissors I woman on top

In this position, the woman scissors the man's head with her legs; this gives the man's penis inside her a tight squeeze and stimulates the woman as well.

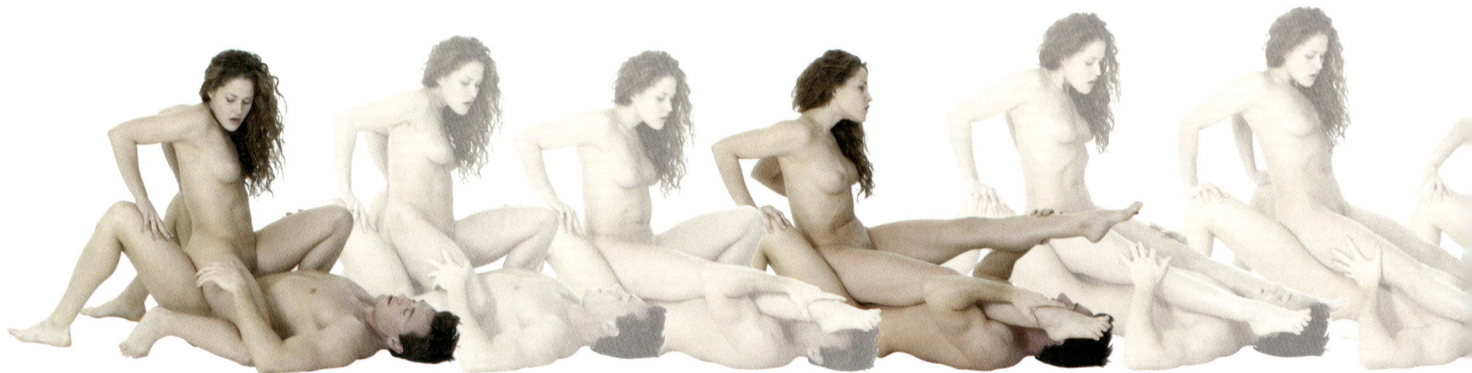

● The man lies down with his knees raised to provide support for his partner. The woman sits astride his waist and leans back against his thighs.

● Once the man has entered her, the woman slowly brings her legs around to the front. As the woman bends her knees to do this, the man sees his penis inside her vagina, which he is likely to find very exciting.

● The man keeps his legs bent so that his partner can lean back on them to keep her balance as she swings her legs straight out in front of her.

● The woman leans backward and rests her hands on the man's knees. This gives her a better grip and makes sure that he stays inside her. The man runs his hands up along her legs to increase her excitement.

visual excitement ▶ **bent legs** ▶ **grip** ▶

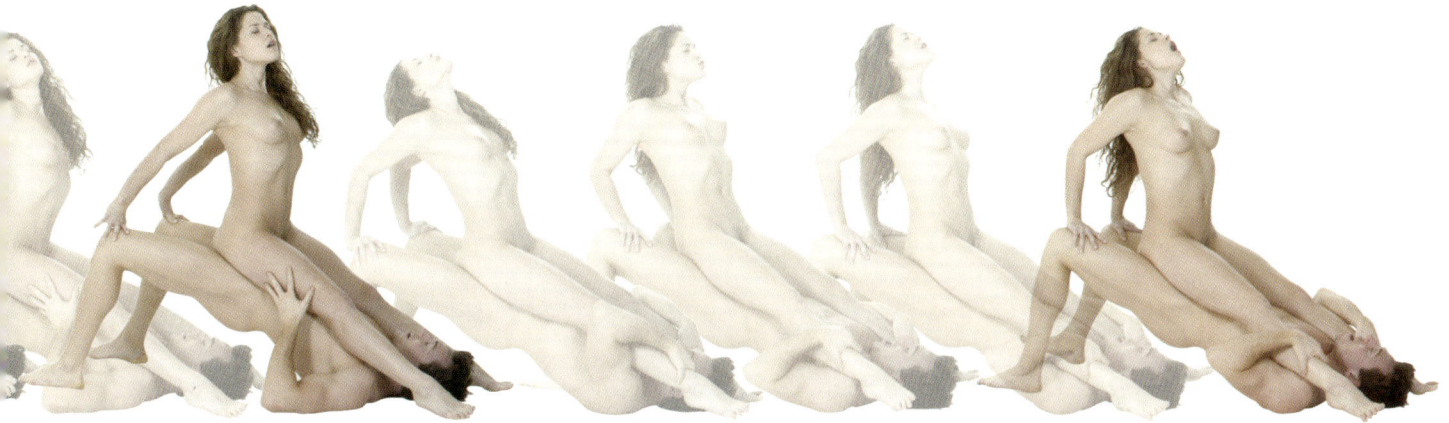

● Pushing her feet against the floor, the woman starts to move up and down on the man's penis while he lowers and raises his hips and thighs. This increases his thrusting capability and intensifies their pleasure.

● The man grips his partner's ankles as the couple rock backward and forward towards their orgasm. If your timing is good, you are likely to reach climax simultaneously.

● Considerable pressure can be achieved if both partners grip firmly. It is an excellent "hard" position if each partner pushes hard against the other to reach orgasm.

● As the man comes, he may thrust so hard as to throw the woman off, so she needs to thrust equally hard downward to stay in position. This helps to intensify the man's orgasm.

thrust ▶ orgasm ▶ use pressure ▶ ‖

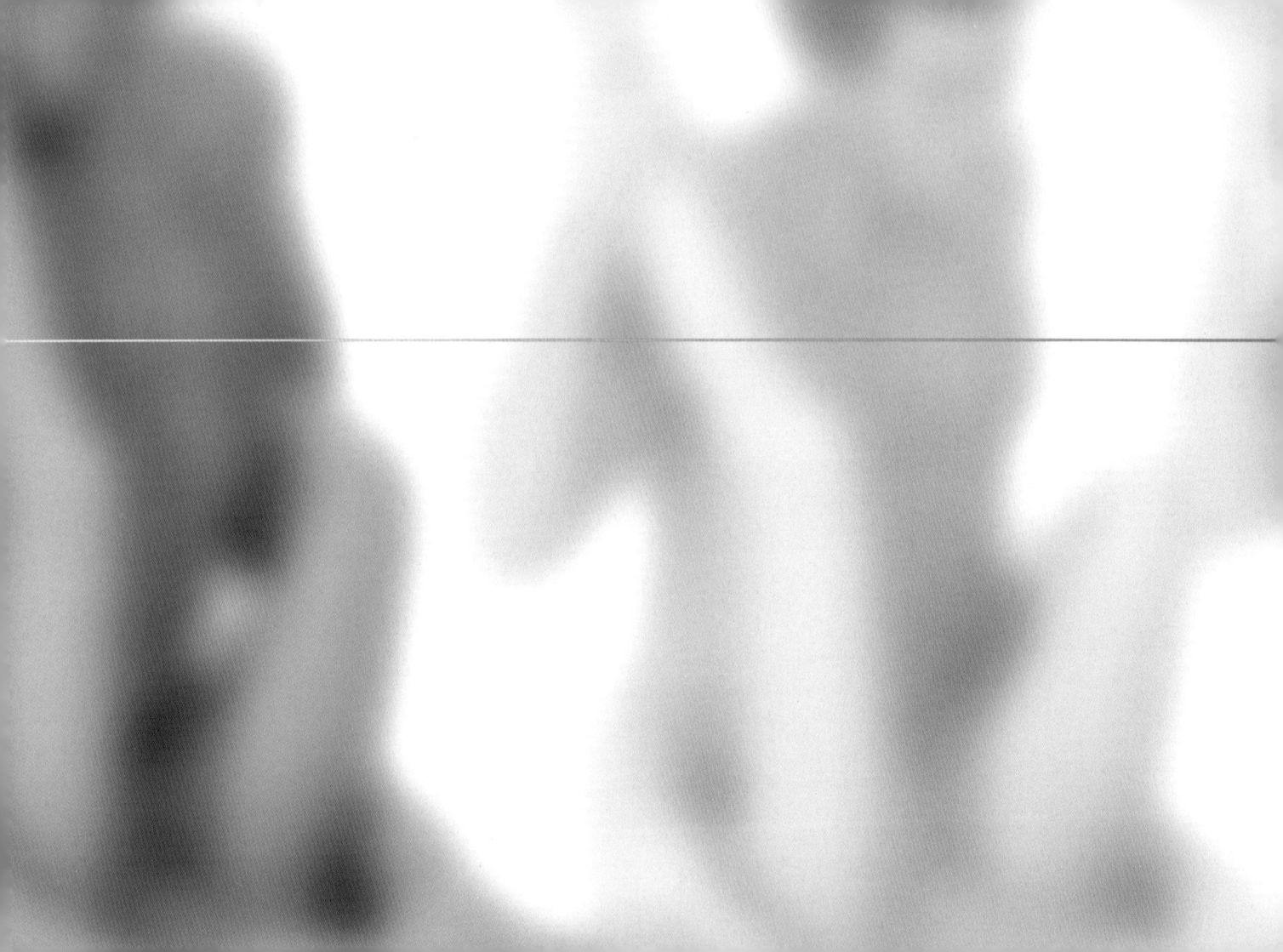

man on top

from oral to man on top

If the man has been pleasuring the woman with his lips and tongue, he might like to maneuver himself carefully into having full sex with her so she can orgasm with him inside her.

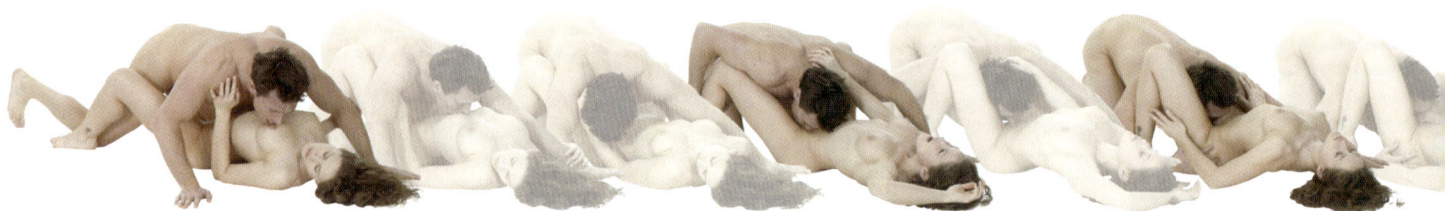

● The woman lies on her back with her knees bent. Supporting his weight on his hands and knees, the man caresses her entire body with his lips and tongue, kissing and licking her.

● As the man works his way down the woman's body, she simply lies back and enjoys the experience of her partner making love to her.

● When the man reaches her vagina, the woman spreads her legs wide to give him easy access. The man positions himself between her legs and licks her clitoris to stimulate her.

● Good oral sex is more than just random licking. Nibble with your lips, push your tongue inside, lick delicately along the sides of the clitoris as well as the perineum, and use your fingers to stimulate the vagina and G spot.

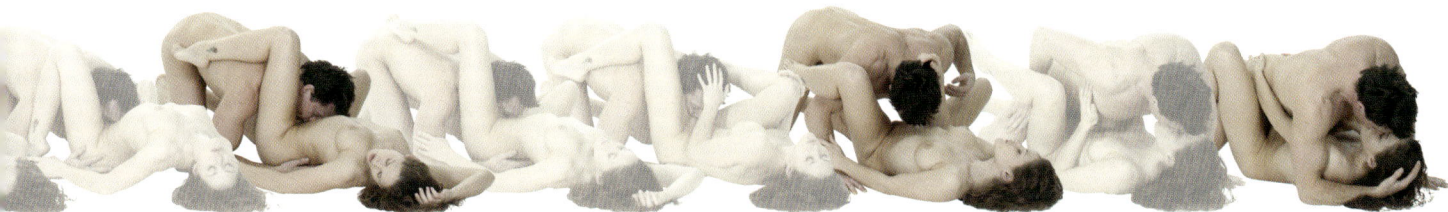

● For deeper penetration, the woman throws her legs over the man's back. This is a very good position for deep oral tongue work.

● As the woman nears orgasm, the man prepares to move up her body. He must make sure that he continues the momentum or the woman will lose her climax.

● The man moves up the woman's body, still masturbating her with his fingers. The woman spreads her legs apart even wider so that she is ready for him to enter her.

● When the man reaches the right position, the woman will be ready for him to slip into her easily. She is likely to reach orgasm almost as soon as he enters her.

scissors II *on top*

Sometimes, when you just want to have rude and raunchy sex, you need a position that gives you a visually arousing experience; one that is athletic, energetic, thrusting, rude, and very naughty.

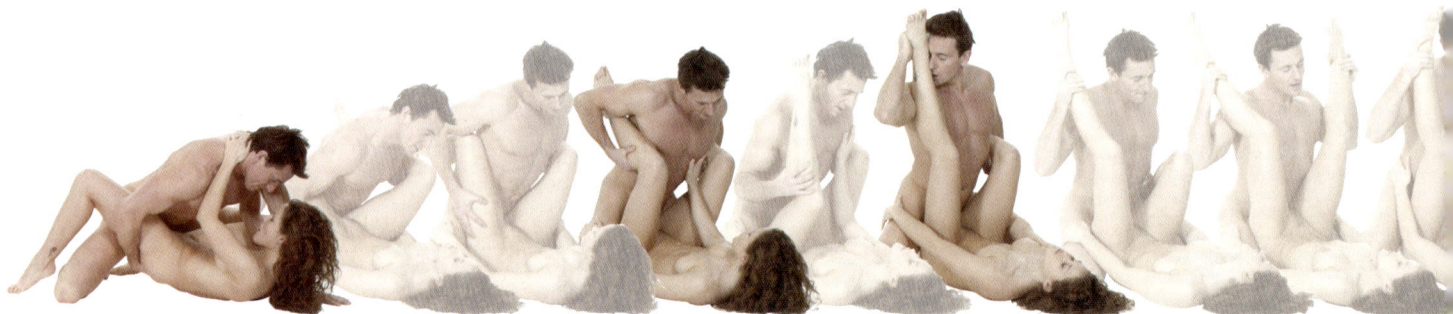

● The couple starts with the woman lying on her back and the man entering her from on top in the classic missionary position. He grips the woman firmly behind her buttocks to pull her hips off the floor.

● Holding on to the man's thighs, the woman forces her hips off the floor and opens her legs to accommodate the man. He pushes hard into her and they maintain eye contact, looking deeply into each other's eyes.

● If the man half kneels, he is able to push very hard. Caressing the woman's legs, he then sits upright to increase the friction on her G spot with his penis inside her.

● As he pushes, the man parts the woman's legs wide so that he can enter her more deeply, more strongly. The woman raises her buttocks to help the man increase his penetration.

■   **push hard**   ▶   **friction**   ▶   ▶

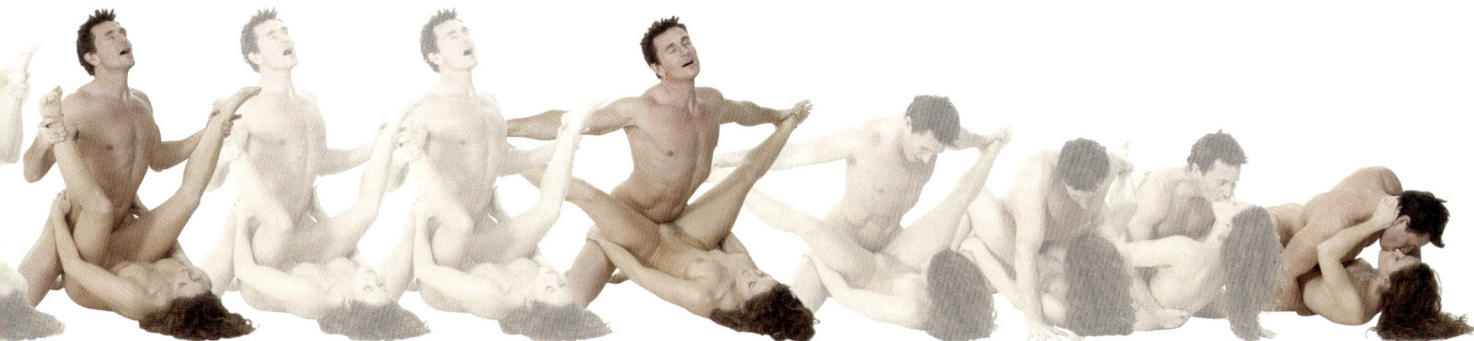

● Moving her hands so as to grip the man firmly around the back of the hips, the woman pulls her partner toward her to increase the friction. The man slowly arches his back as he feels his orgasm nearing.

● As the man reaches orgasm, he spreads the woman's legs even wider to increase his penetration. However, he must take care—she may not be supple enough and such deep penetration may cause her discomfort.

● With the woman's legs spread wide, the man's penis can stimulate her clitoris and G spot simultaneously so that she too may reach orgasm.

● As the couple both come, they will be unable to keep this position for long. Let yourselves collapse into each other's arms. Be close and intimate.

the gymnast

If you are fit and active, healthy, and adventurous, then this is the position for you. It requires a degree of strength, enthusiasm, energy, and creativity.

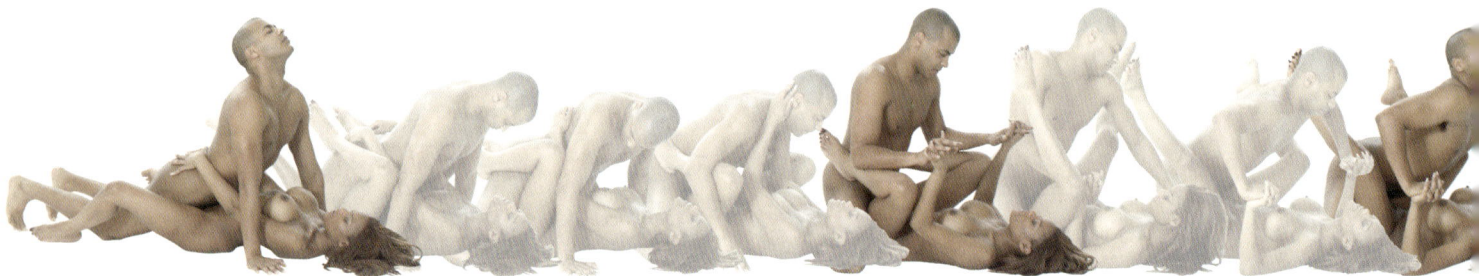

● The man enters the woman, with his legs tucked inside hers. He arches his back and she pulls him tightly to her with a firm hold on his buttocks.

● The woman wraps her legs around the man's back and pulls him to her with her hands on his back. Using his arms to support his weight, the man has the power to make deep, satisfying thrusts into his partner.

● If the man rocks back on his knees, the woman can bring her legs forward while the couple lock hands.

● Pushing down hard on the woman's hands gives the man enough pressure in his groin to thrust quite hard. The woman grips him tightly around his back with her legs.

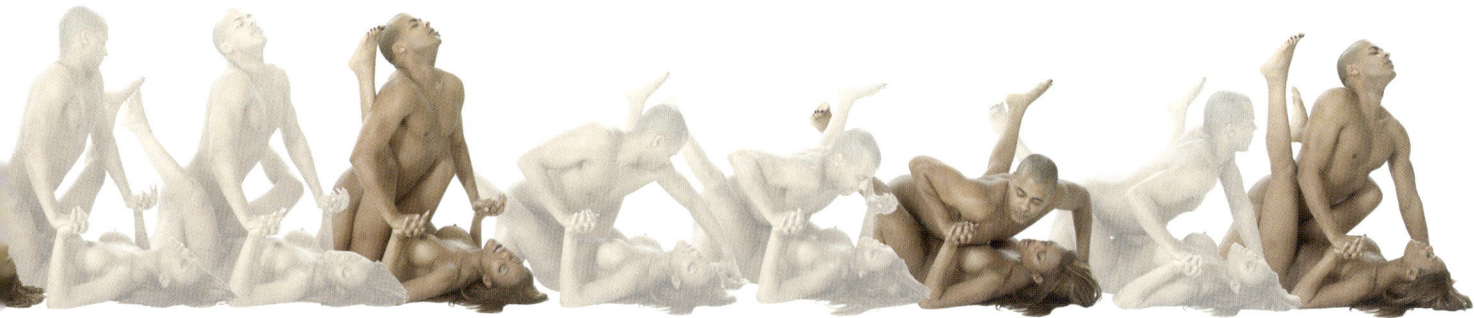

● Although this position does not allow much movement, you will find that it has a fervor and urgency that produce great levels of excitement.

● For greater friction and pressure, the man places one hand flat on the floor next to the woman's head and she grips his hand. Remember to keep eye contact, have fun, laugh at each other, and enjoy yourselves.

● This tends to be a male fantasy position, as it allows the man to orgasm with fierce intensity but does not provide clitoral stimulation. Unless the woman can achieve vaginal orgasm, she is unlikely to climax.

● The man's orgasm can be very intense in this position, especially if the woman grips his buttocks tightly between her legs and squeezes his hand hard as he comes.

▶ enjoy ▶ his orgasm ▶ 11

deeply, madly, truly

In this position the man can achieve maximum penetration, hence the title. If the man has a short penis, this is an excellent position for pleasuring the woman, since it does allow deep entry.

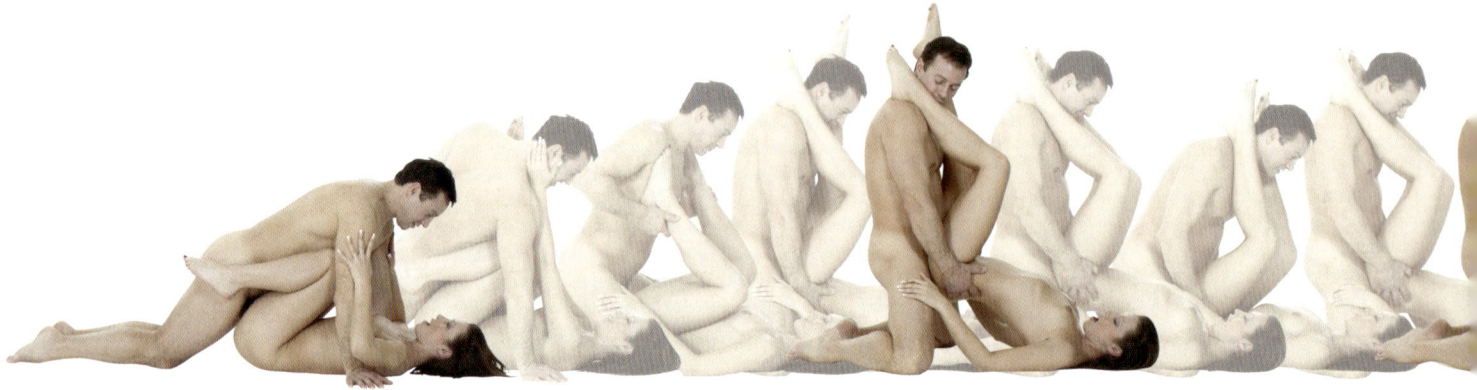

● With the woman lying flat on her back with her knees raised, the man lies on top of her with his legs straight out behind him. As he enters her, the man supports his body weight on his arms, pressing his palms into the floor.

● After warming up with some regular lovemaking, the woman raises her legs, one at a time, and places them against the man's chest with her feet resting either side of his head.

● This position gives the woman a range of leg movements that will determine the depth of her partner's penetration and how much he can thrust against her clitoris.

● By raising her shoulders, the woman changes the angle at which the man enters her. She can adjust her position until she achieves maximum stimulation and satisfaction.

▶ control   ▶ adjust   ▶

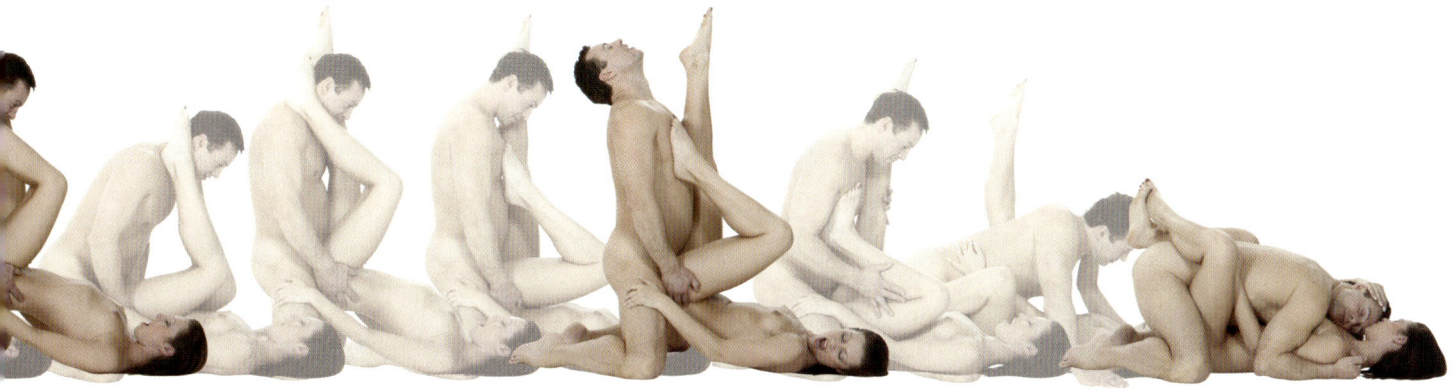

● The man then lifts the woman's hips to gain even greater penetration, and she pulls herself forward as he thrusts against her with her hands on his upper thighs.

● By reaching through the woman's legs, the man can stroke and rub her clitoris to bring her to orgasm. If his timing is good, the couple can reach their orgasms simultaneously.

● As the man comes, the woman pushes hard against his chest with one or both feet while he grips her upper thighs for additional pressure. This is an excellent position for deeply satisfying, hard-thrusting orgasms.

● After the couple have come together, they can collapse easily in this position. The woman wraps her legs around the man as he leans forward to rest on her body. Enjoy being close and intimate.

yogic orgasm

For this position, the woman needs to have practiced yoga and be extremely fit and supple.

If you are confident that you are flexible enough, there is a lot of fun to be had trying this position.

It is always good—and healthy—to laugh during sex.

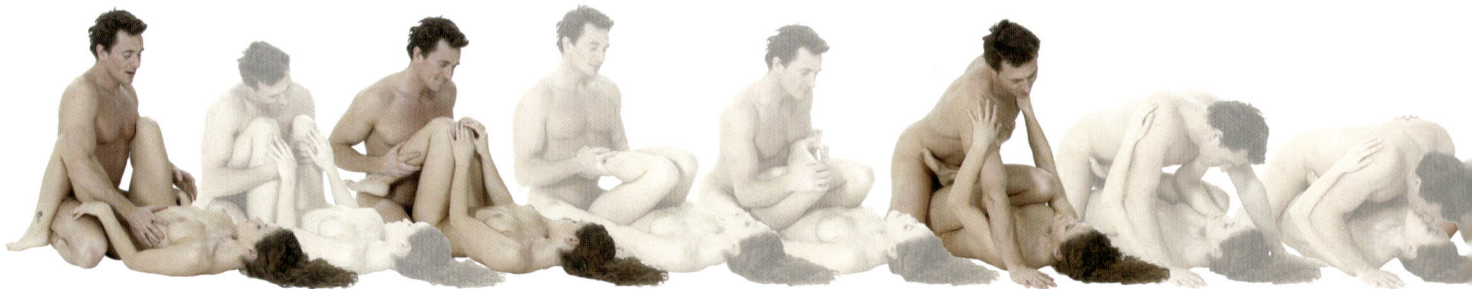

● The woman lies on the floor with her knees raised. Kneeling between her legs, the man caresses his partner's breasts and stimulates her clitoris before entering her.

● To further her excitement, he strokes her legs while she strokes his hands as they move across her body. The man can enter the woman's vagina or her anus.

● Once he has entered the woman, the man folds her legs into his chest and grips her knees firmly. This enables him to thrust harder and stronger.

● With his partner's legs still folded, the man leans forward and kisses the woman. Penetration will not be very deep in this position, but the man's penis will stimulate the woman's clitoris and allow her to climax.

stroke ▶ thrust ▶ orgasm ▶

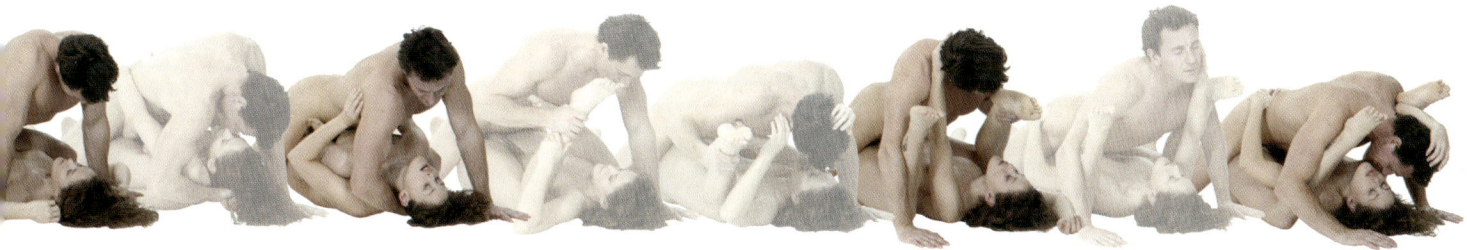

● If she is supple, the woman can open her legs fairly wide and keep her knees bent. This enables the man to enter her more deeply. He can also put his hand behind her neck to pull her toward his chest.

● By holding the woman's leg, the man gains better purchase for his thrusts and is still able to kiss her. Kissing is important while making love because it keeps the intimacy going.

● Just before orgasm, the woman can put her knees on the floor on either side of her body. The man can then alternate his thrusts between deep and shallow to further her excitement.

● If the woman is very supple, she will be able to put her ankles over her partner's shoulders. This is a very good position in which to achieve very deep penetration, if desired.

the missionary *man on top*

The story goes that when the first European missionaries reached the South Sea Islands, they were spied on by the locals to see if their lovemaking was any different. Since the couples happened to be using this position, it became known as "The Missionary" and the name stuck.

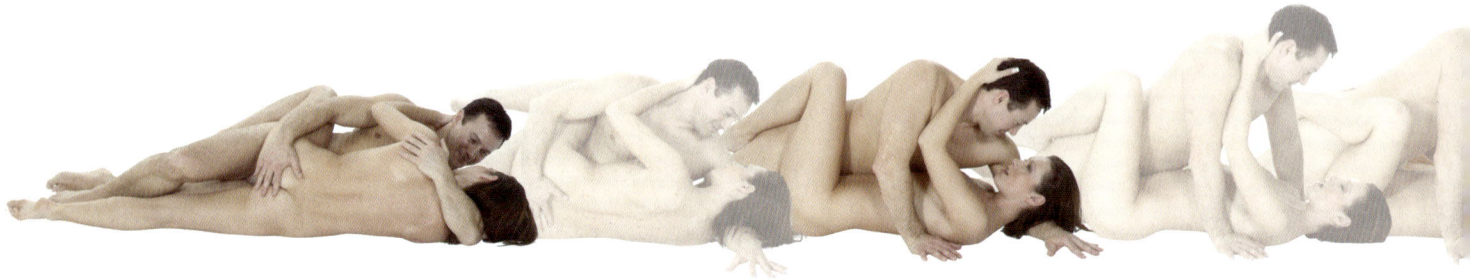

- The man does not have to be lying on top of the woman in this position. You can make love lying on your side, facing each other. Start in this way and embrace.

- The man rolls on top of the woman and pulls her underneath him at the same time. The woman places one leg over his back to let him enter her and guides him onto her body.

- The woman wraps her legs around the man's back and pulls him tightly to her chest. She could also open her legs wide to receive him. This is a very intimate position, loving and close.

- The man take his weight on his arms to avoid crushing his partner. The woman reaches up to caress his face while he is making love to her.

▶ **be intimate** ▶ **caress** ▶

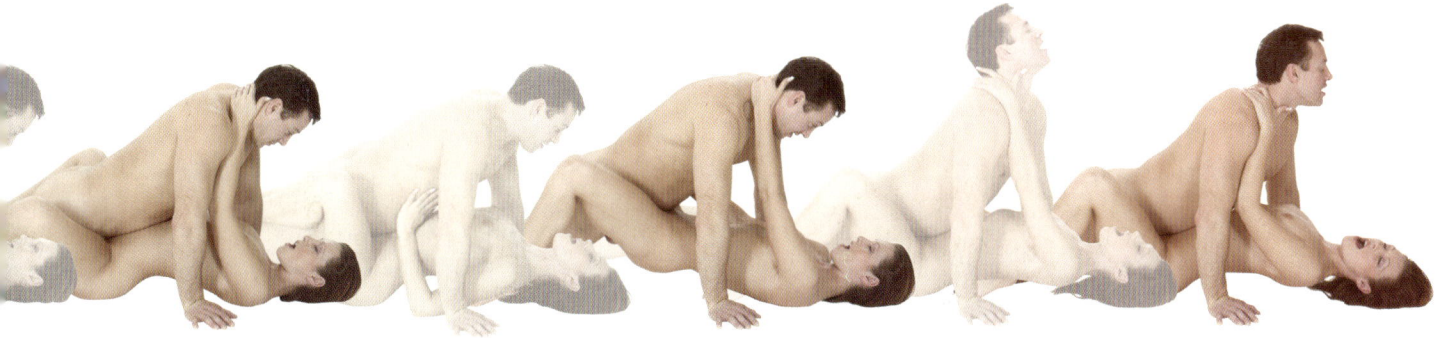

● As the man thrusts into her, the woman thrusts upward with her hips and pulls down hard on his neck to pull him to her. Maintain eye contact throughout to keep it sexy.

● For deeper penetration, the woman arches her back so that her pubic bone is pushed upward against his, which stimulates her clitoris.

● In her passion, the woman pushes her hips off the ground and thrusts hard against the man. Timing his thrusts with hers, the man ensures that they climax simultaneously, if that is what they both want.

● The woman caresses the man's chest and squeezes his nipples hard as she comes while he thrusts hard against her, making sure his pubic bone remains in contact with hers to help her reach orgasm.

eye contact   ▶   stimulate   ▶   orgasm   ▶   ❚❚

pivots

man on top

Timing, strength, and coordination are needed for pivots, together with stamina. Basically, the woman hangs on the man's neck while he rocks them to their orgasm, but the results are tremendous fun and great sex. If the man suffers from a neck injury, however, he should avoid attempting this position.

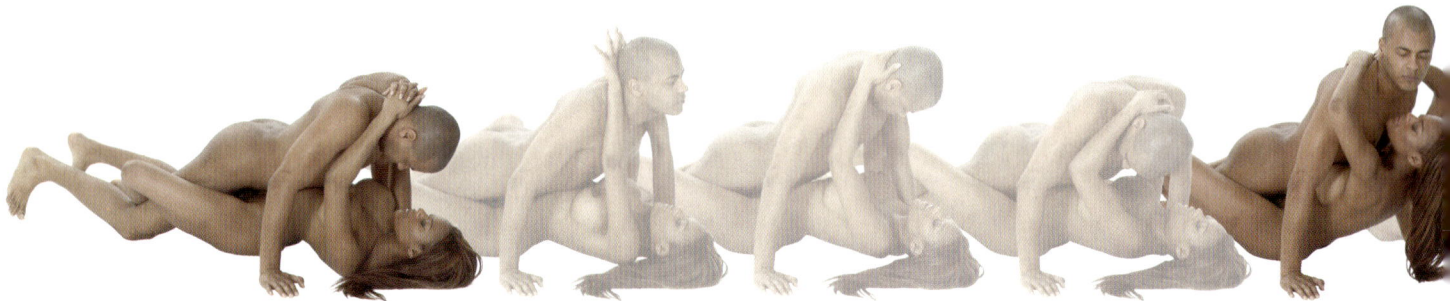

● The couple starts in the traditional missionary position, with the man on top and the woman underneath lying on her back. The woman entwines her legs around the man's.

● The woman reaches up to clasp her hands behind the man's neck as he takes his weight on his arms and gets ready to thrust upward.

● As the man pulls upward, he takes the woman with him, pivoted on his neck. There is little stimulation in this position, but it is very exciting as it is intimate and very close.

● If the man is very strong, he can lever himself upward quite some distance, taking the woman with him. The couple rock to and fro in this position until the man tires.

■   entwine   ▶   be intimate   ▶   rock to and fro   ▶

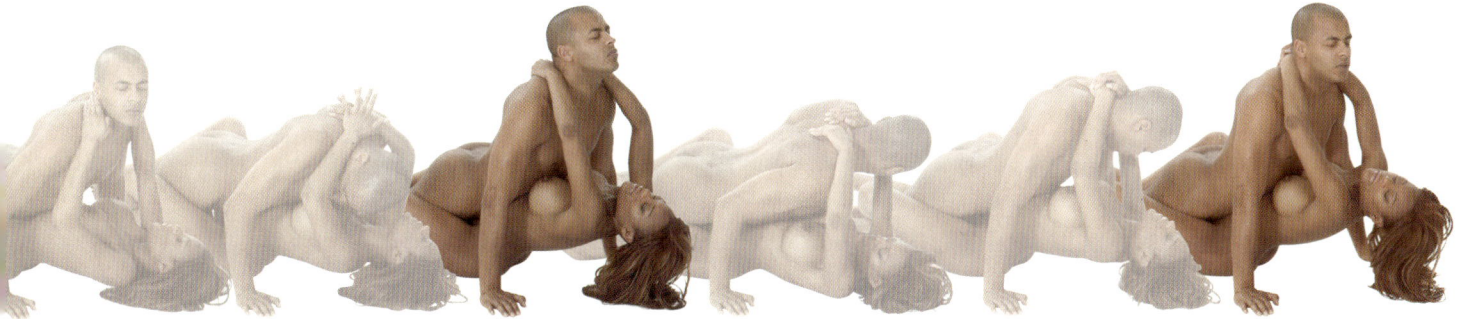

- As he rocks backward, the woman can arch her back and press her breasts against him, and he can kiss her and suck her nipples.

- By arching his back as he rocks, the man enters the woman more deeply. As he straightens his back, his thrusts become even more vigorous.

- Twisting is tiring but great fun. If the man twists his body from side to side, the action twists his penis, which, in turn, stimulates the internal walls of the woman's vagina.

- As the man reaches his orgasm, the woman should go limp and hang on his neck. The man continues to support his weight on his arms.

splayed *on top*

If the woman likes deep penetration she will enjoy this position, but it requires a considerable degree of litheness and flexibility. It can also be quite tough on the man's back, so he needs to be strong and not suffer from any back injuries.

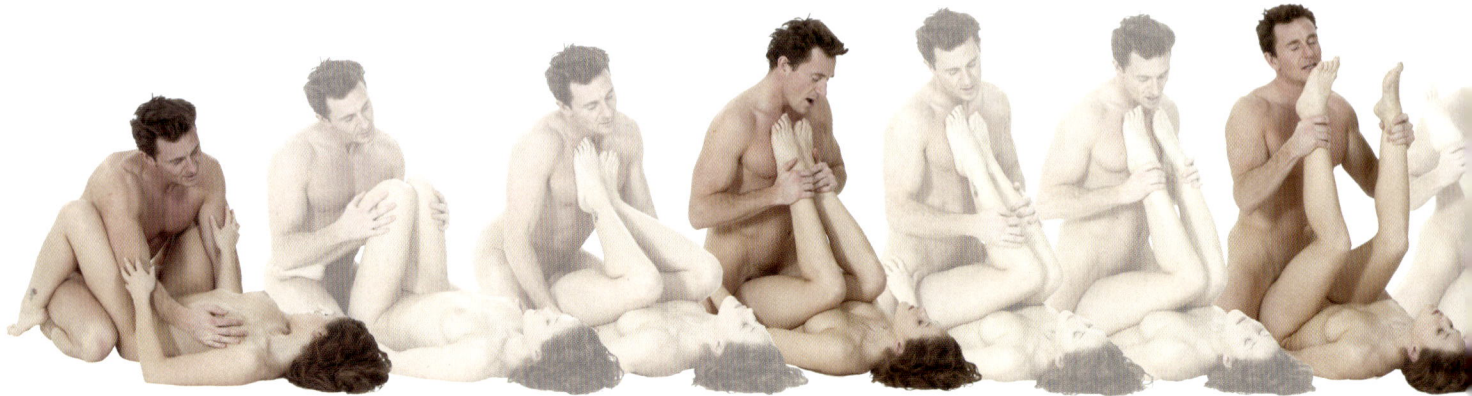

● The woman lies on her back with her knees raised and the man kneels between her legs. At this stage he does not need to enter her but can caress her and stroke her breasts.

● The man strokes the woman all over and caresses her legs and vulva. As her excitement increases, the man prepares to enter her. She raises her legs to accommodate him, placing her feet lightly on his chest.

● As he enters his partner, the man holds her ankles, which provides a thrill for both of them. The woman reaches down to caress his hips and thighs.

● As he thrusts into her, the man pushes down hard on her legs and she presses her palms into the floor. The man supports himself on the woman's legs as he makes love to her.

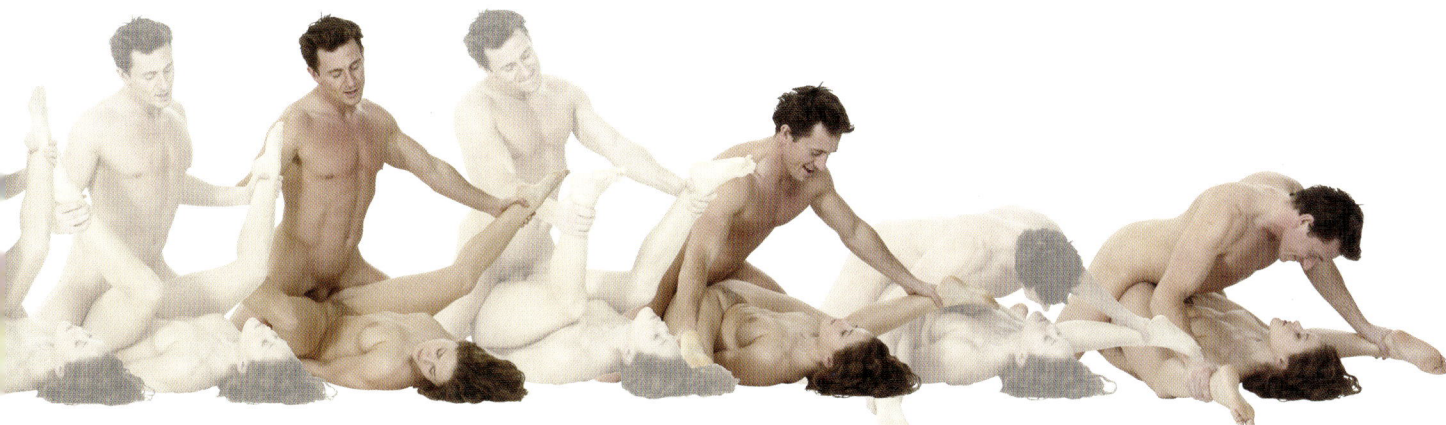

● By spreading the woman's legs apart, the man can watch his penis sliding in and out of her, which is visually exciting for most men. He also reaches down to stroke his partner's clitoris as he watches.

● During sex it is important to have fun, so remember to talk to each other, laugh, and even tell jokes. Sex does not have to be all serious.

● If the woman is very supple, the man can widen her legs further to give very deep penetration indeed.

● The ultimate position, if the woman is supple enough, is for her to place her feet on the floor at either side of her head. This allows the man to penetrate her deeply.

loving position

In this position the couple can enjoy themselves intimately, be close and loving, and caress and stroke each other to climax. This is a position for a man and a woman who are very much in love.

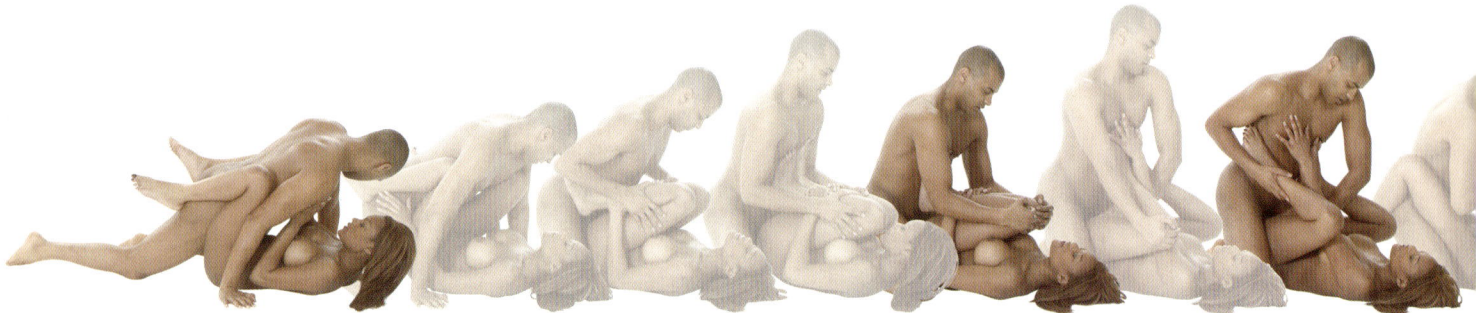

● The couple make love with the woman lying on her back and her legs wrapped around the man's back. The man enters her and supports his body weight on his arms.

● The woman raises her knees and the man alters his position to give her maximum satisfaction.

● The woman folds her legs to give the man deep penetration and reaches up to stroke his chest and nipples, increasing his excitement. He reaches through her legs to stroke her vulva and further her excitement.

● As the man reaches through to stroke the woman's clitoris, she reaches to stroke his penis. The man slides slowly in and out of her. As their fingers meet in the wetness of sex, the sensation can be extremely erotic.

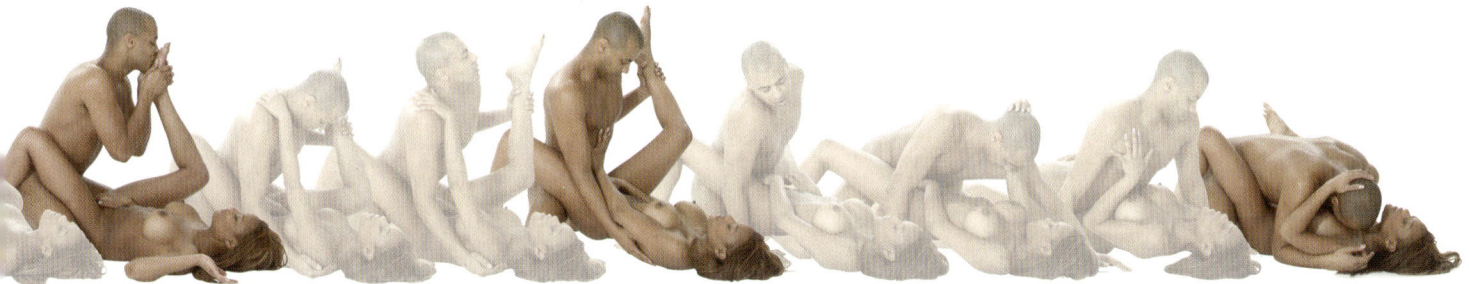

● If she wants to, the woman can masturbate herself. While she does this, the man licks and sucks her toes. Take the time to stroke and love each other in this position.

● The man lifts the woman up by her buttocks so he can enter her more deeply. He watches her masturbating as he thrusts gently into her.

● The woman masturbates herself to orgasm in this position, and, with skill, the man can hold back until she is in the throes of her orgasm. He then thrusts rapidly and strongly into her and comes at the same time.

● As the couple both come and collapse in their exhaustion, they can relax into a loving and intimate embrace and fall asleep in each other's arms.

don't rush ▶ watch ▶ be skillful ▶ 11

pleasuring the woman

Sometimes it is good for the man to delay or even postpone his orgasm so he can concentrate entirely on pleasuring the woman. The skillful and experienced lover receives his pleasure by giving his lover pleasure without seeking to satisfy his own needs.

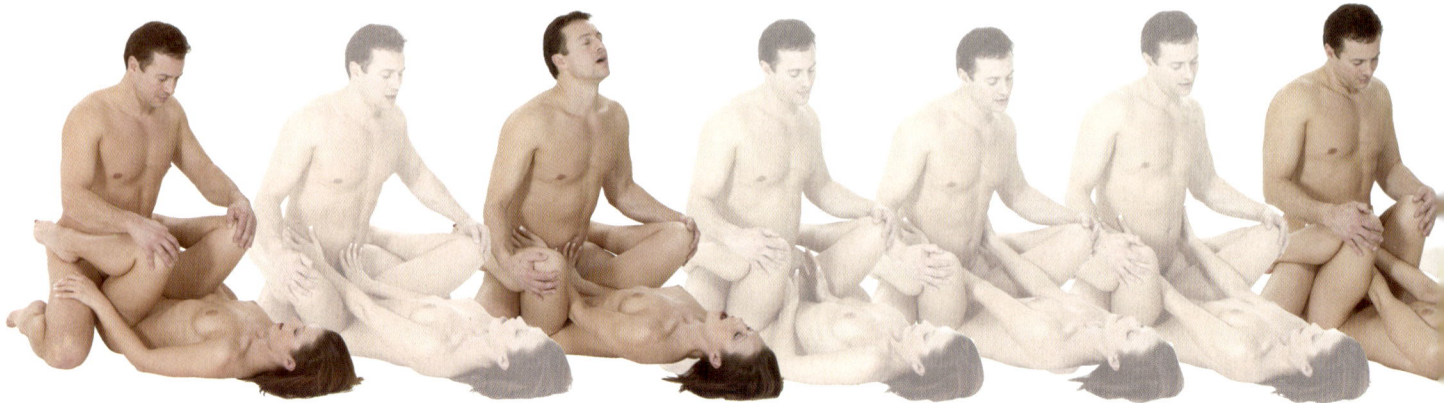

● As the woman prepares herself to be pleasured, she adopts whatever position she likes and feels comfortable in. Here, the woman has chosen to lie back to enjoy herself.

● The man kneels inside the woman's legs and enters her. He inserts his penis very gently, very slowly, and very teasingly. If he does nine shallow thrusts and then one deep thrust, the man will excite the woman wildly.

● At the same time, the woman strokes the man, caresses his penis as it is pulled out from her vagina, and masturbates herself. Whatever turns her on; this is her time, her treat.

● The woman should set the pace and tone for this lovemaking session. Does she want it fast and furious? Or slow and lingering? It is entirely up to her, and the experienced, skillful man will go along with whatever she wants.

■   **shallow thrusts** ▶   **be indulgent** ▶   **control** ▶

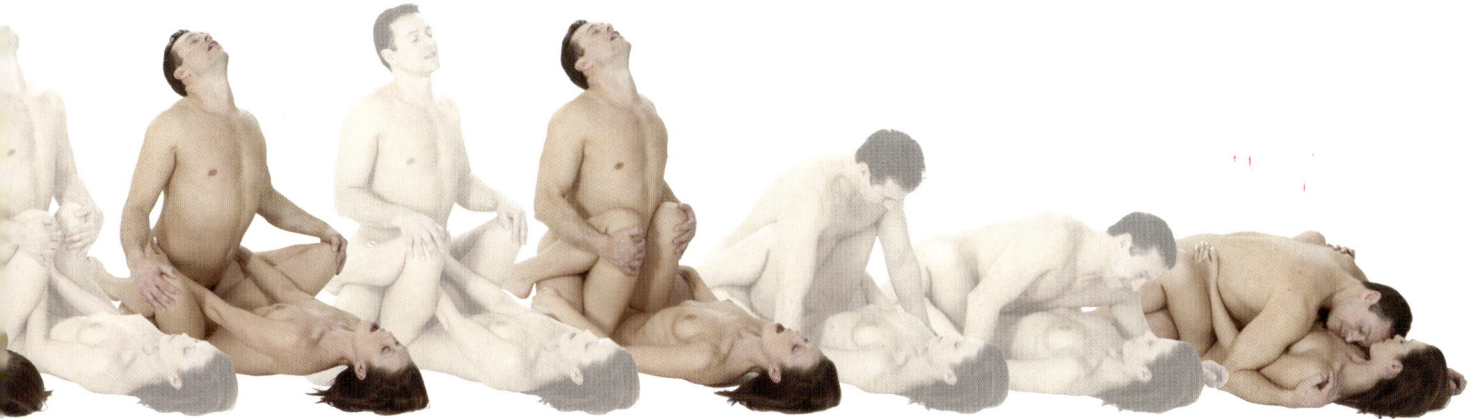

● This does not mean that the lovemaking should be mechanical or stilted. Quite the reverse, in fact. The man should be passionate, abandoned, and wild. He is simply concentrating on her orgasm rather than his own.

● The man squeezes her legs, strokes her vigorously, moans, groans, and excites her to express his passion. He lets the woman set the pace, tell him what she wants, and then he responds to her every need.

● If the woman is reluctant to shout out her needs, then she can use her body to express herself, making pleasurable noises when the man satisfies her desires.

● If the woman wants to be held close, be intimate, and loving, then that is fine. The man does whatever she wants, holding and cuddling her as much and as long as she needs.

be passionate ▶ **respond** ▶ **express yourself** ▶ II

pleasuring the man

Men have had to become skillful, considerate, and courteous lovers over the last few decades.
It is no longer acceptable for the man to orgasm, roll over, and go to sleep. But if the woman has
already been satisfied and wishes to continue making love, it is all right for him to please himself.

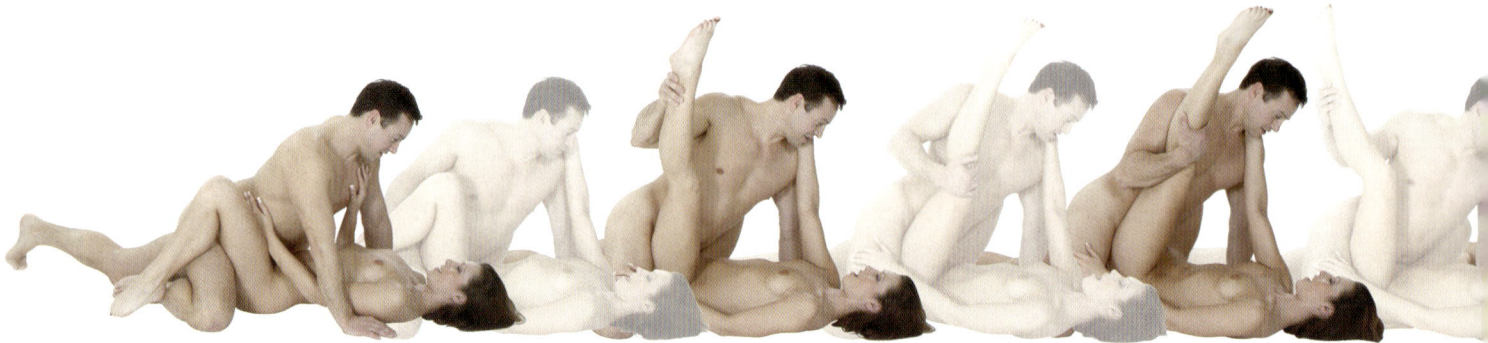

● The woman lies down on her back and the man, positioned between her legs, enters her. She has already come and is feeling sexy and very ready for her man to come inside her.

● The man takes his time enjoying being inside her and not feeling any pressure to satisfy her, since he has already done that in some other way. This exercise is for him and him alone.

● He enjoys playing with his partner, getting her to lift one leg to see what it feels like, to change the pressure on his penis inside her, and to experiment with the sensation she is receiving.

● He experiments with the speed and strength of his thrusts and enjoys making love to her without worrying about making her come. He can concentrate on his own sensations.

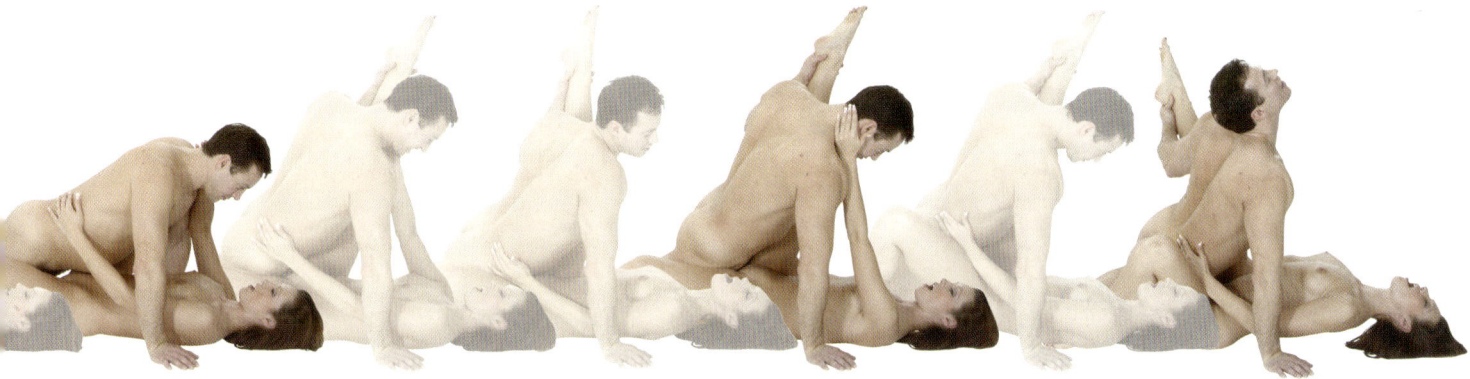

● The woman uses her hands on his hips to pull him to her. She whispers that she loves the feeling of him inside her, which excites him. She keeps eye contact and smiles a lot to reassure him that this is good.

● When the man feels his orgasm beginning to rise, he slows down, since he does not want to come too quickly. He is enjoying this sensation, enjoying making love slowly and sensuously with his partner.

● The woman thrusts up against the man to excite him more and he can wait no longer as his orgasm builds up. He thrusts harder and faster, stronger and deeper. She senses his orgasm is close and moans to stimulate him.

● As he comes, the man lets himself go, making as much noise as he wants. He shouts and moans, exciting his partner, and she too comes again. He collapses onto her, exhausted, satisfied both physically and emotionally.

experimenting *man on top*

Sometimes it is fun to throw caution to the wind, let your hair down, and just do whatever you want. At other times it is helpful to follow a set technique. Lovemaking can be wild or controlled, passionate or loving. Sometimes it can be all of these things at once.

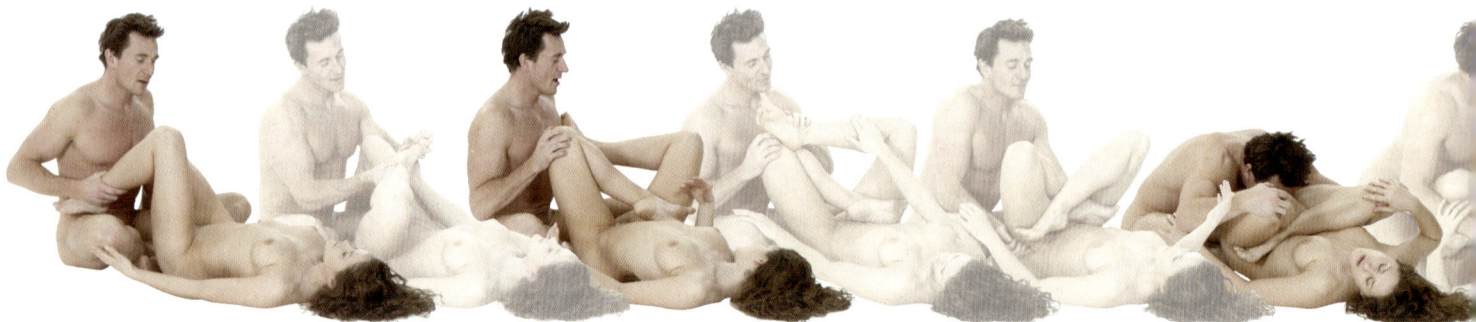

● In this exercise, you can follow whatever turns you on. The couple start caressing each other with the woman lying on her back and the man sitting between her legs with his fingers inside her stimulating her.

● If she can do so, the woman decides it would be fun to cross her legs and lie in a lotus position so that the man can gain better access to her. He likes the idea and wants to join her in the experiment.

● The man helps the woman into this position and finds he can insert several fingers while using his other hand to masturbate her. The woman likes this and gets very excited and moist.

● The man realizes that he can lean forward to give her oral sex, so he inserts his tongue and licks inside her vagina. By now the woman is very excited and asks him to make love.

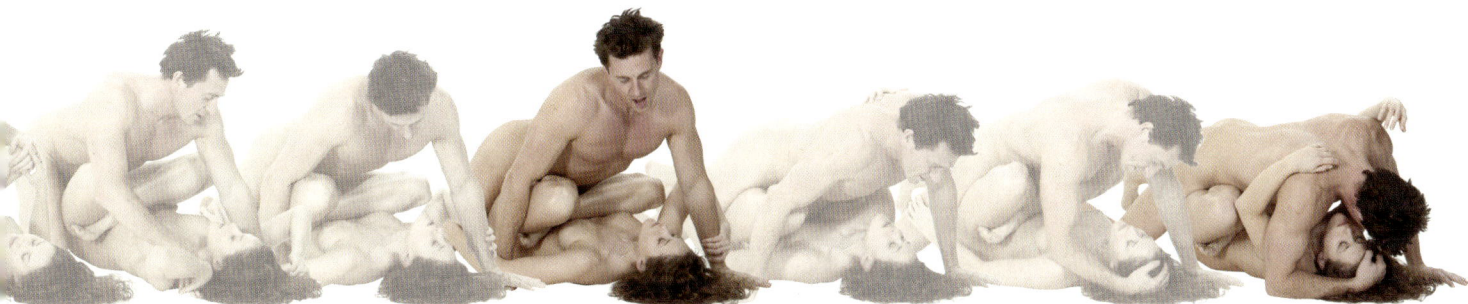

● The woman stays in the same position while the man maneuvers himself so that he can enter her. He teases her by not sliding his penis completely into her but by using the head of it to stroke her clitoris.

● The woman begs him to insert his penis properly so she can feel his entire length inside her and he is happy to oblige. As he enters her he takes his weight on his arms.

● The man thrusts slowly at first and then faster as she eggs him on and moans for him to come inside her. She feels her own orgasm approaching and he times it so that he holds back until she is reaching climax.

● The woman loses herself in her orgasm and the man comes too. By experimenting, the couple have found a new way of making love. They might not use it often, but they have learned more about their desires and needs.

index

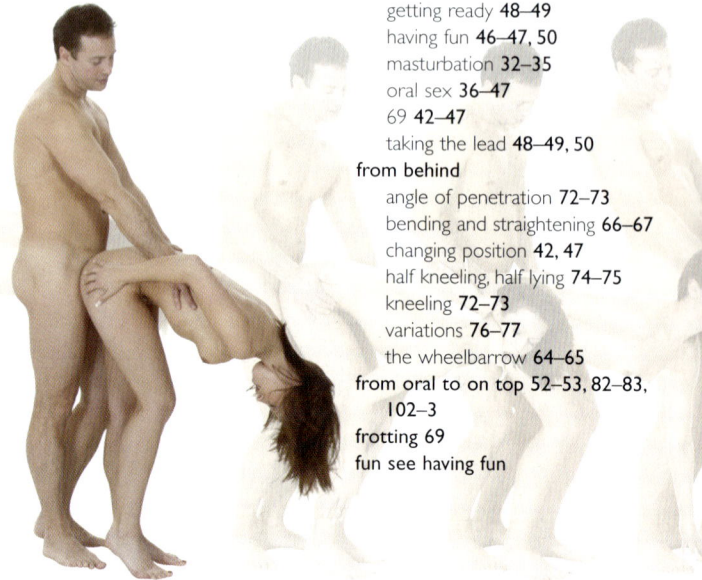

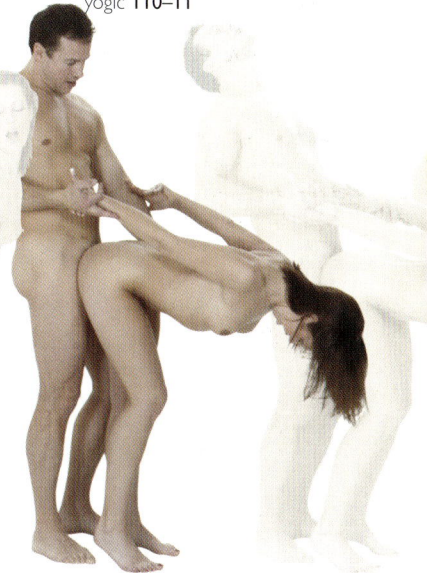

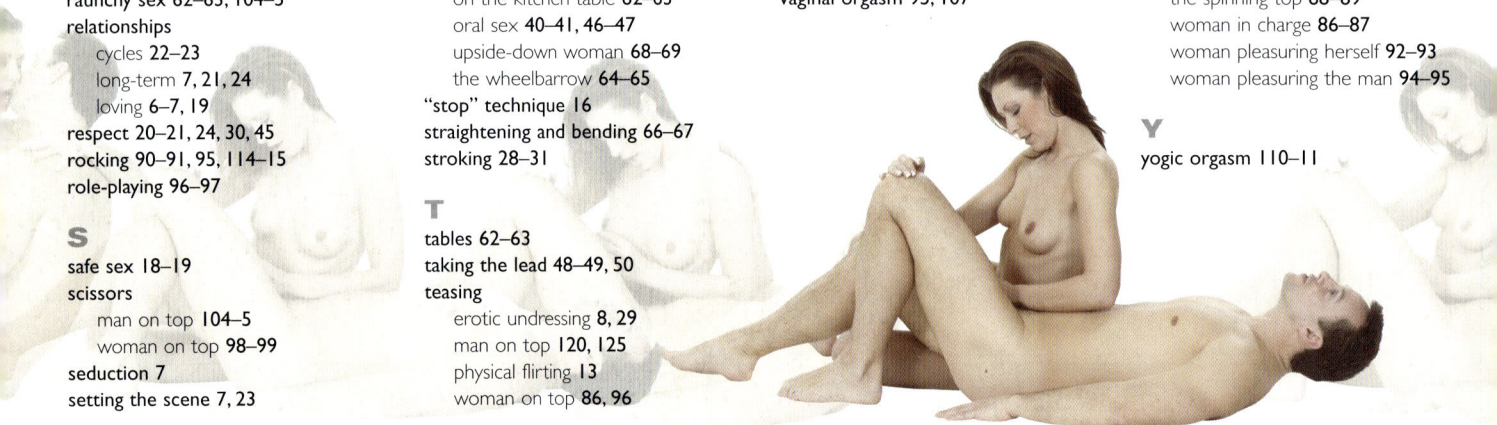